VEGGIE AND PROTEIN

Cookbook

By CYNTHIA LEONARD

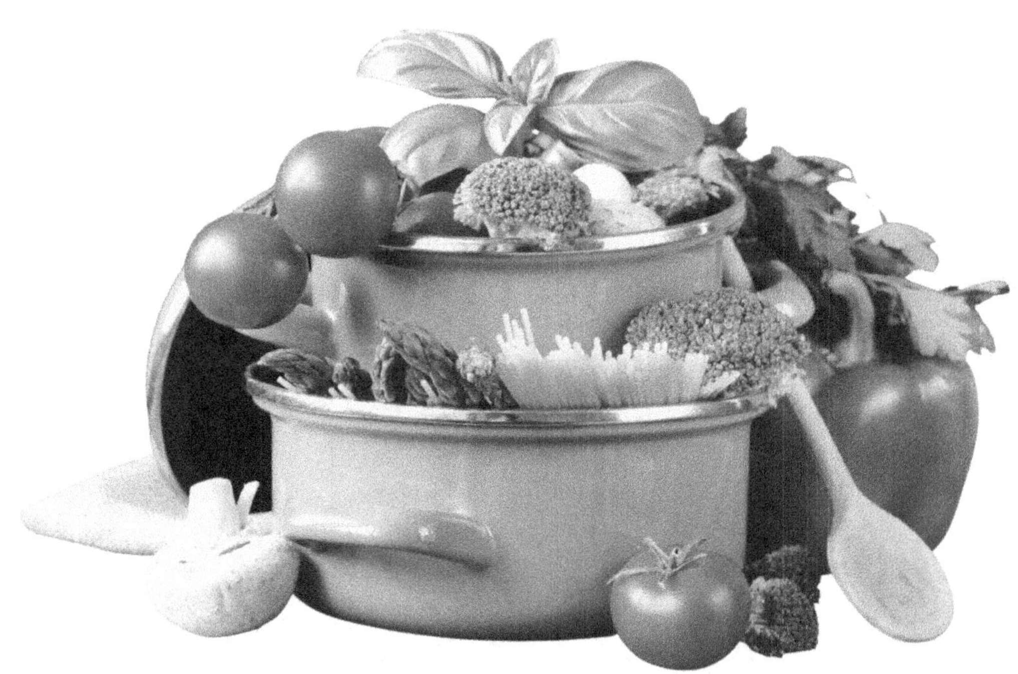

TABLE OF CONTENTS

ABOUT THIS COOKBOOK

Here it is - the **"Veggie and Protein Cookbook."** Every page of this delectable collection offers a harmonic balance of flavour and nutrition as it celebrates colourful plant-based components that are expertly combined with a range of protein sources. This cookbook promises to uplift and inspire your meals, regardless of your level of culinary expertise. It offers a wide variety of dishes that not only tempt the senses but also support a well-balanced, high-protein lifestyle. Take a culinary adventure that demonstrates that eating healthily can be tasty and satisfying, from creative vegetarian meals to protein-packed treats. Prepare to learn the art of creating wholesome, tasty meals and delve into a world of delicious combinations with the versatile Cookbook.

Benefits of Veggie and Protein-rich Diet

Numerous health advantages may be obtained from a diet high in veggies and protein. Here are a few main benefits:

DENSITY OF NUTRIENTS

Carrots: Rich in vital vitamins, minerals and antioxidants, carrots support general health and wellbeing.

Proteins: Meals high in protein provide the amino acids required for the body's upkeep, development and repair.

Controlling Weight

Veggies: Rich in fibre and low in calories, veggies may help you feel fuller and control your weight.

Proteins: Foods high in protein also help with satiety, which lowers calorie intake overall and aids in weight reduction or maintenance.

Growth and Repair of Muscles

Proteins: Necessary for maintaining, repairing, and growing muscle. Sufficient protein consumption is essential for bodybuilders, sportsmen, and those who exercise often.

Regulation of Blood Sugar

Vegetables: Vegetables' high fibre content lowers the risk of diabetes by regulating blood sugar levels.

Proteins: Including protein with meals helps reduce blood sugar rises and help stabilise blood sugar levels.

Heart Conditions

Vegetables: Because of their high fibre and potassium content, certain vegetables, such leafy greens, are linked to a decreased risk of cardiovascular illnesses.

Proteins: Certain protein sources, such as nuts, lentils and fatty fish, are good for the heart and may help decrease cholesterol.
gastrointestinal health

Heart Conditions

Veggies: Packed in fibre, veggies help maintain a healthy gut microbiome and avoid constipation.
Proteins: Enough protein in a diet that is well-balanced may help maintain good digestive health.

Enhanced Immune Response

Veggies: Some veggies, including broccoli and bell peppers, are rich in antioxidants and vitamin C, which help to strengthen the immune system.

Proteins: A sufficient diet of proteins is necessary for the synthesis of antibodies and other immune system components.

Bone Well-being

Veggies: Calcium is essential for healthy bones and may be found in some veggies, such as broccoli and kale.

Proteins: Protein is essential for preserving bone mass and warding off diseases like osteoporosis.

Vegetables: Eating a diet high in vegetables is linked to a decreased chance of developing chronic illnesses, such as certain malignancies.

Proteins: Getting enough protein may help keep muscles from withering away and preserve general health, which lowers the chance of developing a number of ailments.

CONTROLLING APPETITE AND SATIETY

Vegetables: Vegetables' high fibre content helps regulate appetite by promoting feelings of fullness.

Proteins: Foods high in protein also help you feel fuller and less likely to overeat.

Diversity and balance in your diet are essential. A broad range of nutrients necessary for optimum health may be obtained by combining different types of vegetables with different protein sources.

Tips for Incorporating More Vegetables and Proteins into Your Meals

Increasing the amount of veggies and proteins in your diet is a fantastic method to improve its nutritional content. *Here are some pointers to assist you in doing this:*

VEGETABLES

❖ To guarantee you get a wide variety of nutrients, including a variety of veggies in your diet.

❖ To make meals interesting, try experimenting with diverse flavours, textures, and colours.

Prepare Meals:

Prepare and stock veggies ahead of time to provide convenient and speedy access during peak hours.

For usage throughout the week, think about preparing a large quantity of roasted or grilled veggies.

Mix Into Smoothies:

❖ To add even more nutrients to your morning smoothies, including leafy greens like kale or spinach.

❖ To add extra nutrients to sauces or soups, try mixing veggies.

Replace Grains with Veggies:

Use vegetable substitutes in lieu of typical grains, such as zucchini noodles or cauliflower rice.

Smart Snack:

Store chopped vegetables in the refrigerator for easy access to snacks. Serve them with guacamole, hummus or yoghurt-based dips.

Keep Them Out of Recipes:

Add finely chopped or grated veggies to casseroles, spaghetti sauces and meatloaf recipes.

PROTEIN

Sources of Lean Protein:

Select lean protein sources such as turkey, chicken breast, fish, tofu, lentils and low-fat dairy.

Plant-Based Proteins:

Increase the amount of plant-based protein in your meals by including items like almonds, quinoa, edamame, beans and lentils.

Methods of Preparation:

Instead of frying, use healthy cooking techniques like grilling, baking, steaming or sautéing.

Breakfast Packed with Protein:

Eat a breakfast high in protein, such as eggs, Greek yoghurt or a smoothie made with protein powder.

Eat a Protein Snack:

Between meals, munch on items high in protein, such as nuts, seeds, Greek yoghurt or cottage cheese to stay full.

Increase Your Protein Intake:

Use protein to enhance your meals by adding it to side dishes like chickpea-based recipes or quinoa salad.

Conscientious Portion Management:

To make sure you're getting enough protein without going overboard, pay attention to portion sizes.

Overall Advice:

Arrange Well-Balanced Meals:

At every meal, try to strike a balance between nutritious grains, proteins, veggies and healthy fats.

Try Different Herbs & Spices:

Use herbs and spices to flavour food instead of adding too much sugar, salt or harmful condiments.

Maintain Hydration:

For the sake of your general health and digestion, sip on plenty of water throughout the day.

Gradual Modifications:

To help your taste receptors acclimatise and to make the changeover more durable, introduce these modifications gradually.

A healthy and well-balanced diet may be achieved over time by making little, regular adjustments. Pay attention to your body and choose what suits your tastes and way of life the best.

APPETISERS AND SNACKS

Spinach and Artichoke Stuffed Mushrooms

Ingredients:

- 16 big button mushrooms with their stems removed and cleaned
- One tablespoon of olive oil
- One little onion, diced finely
- 2 minced garlic cloves
- One cup of thawed frozen chopped spinach *with extra water squeezed out*
- One cup of chopped canned artichoke hearts
- Grated Parmesan cheese, 1/2 a cup
- 1/2 a cup of cream cheese
- To taste, add salt and pepper.
- Half a cup of breadcrumbs, *optional for garnish*
- Chopped fresh parsley *(for garnish)*

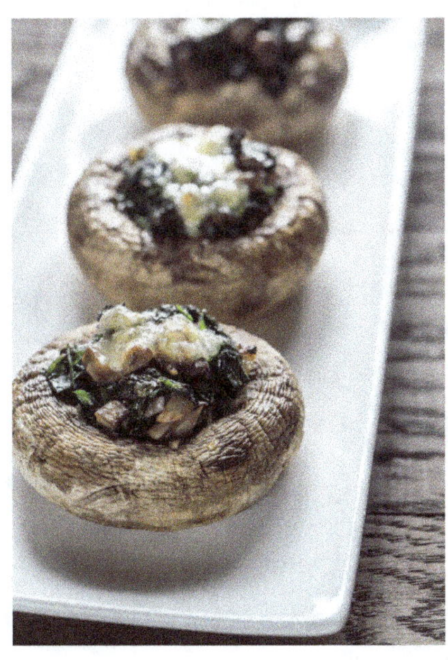

Guidelines:

Turn the oven on to 375°F, or 190°C.

Take off the stems and clean the mushrooms. The mushroom caps should be put on a baking pan.

Heat the olive oil in a pan over medium heat. When the onions are transparent, add the chopped onions and sauté.

Once aromatic, add the minced garlic to the pan and sauté it for an additional one to two minutes.

Add the chopped spinach and simmer for a further two to three minutes or until well cooked.

Simmer the chopped artichoke hearts in the pan for a further two to three minutes.

The sautéed veggies should be combined with cream cheese and Parmesan cheese in a mixing basin. Blend until well blended. To taste, add salt and pepper for seasoning.

Fill each mushroom cap to the brim with the spinach and artichoke mixture.

For a crunchy texture, you may choose to add breadcrumbs to the top of the packed mushrooms.

Bake for 20 to 25 minutes in a preheated oven or until the filling is bubbling and brown and the mushrooms are soft.

Take out of the oven and sprinkle with freshly cut parsley.

These Stuffed Mushrooms with Spinach and Artichoke make a delicious appetiser or party snack.

Quinoa and Black Bean Sliders

Ingredients

For the Sliders:
- One cup of cooked quinoa

- One can (15 oz) of rinsed and drained black beans
- Half a cup of breadcrumbs *(if necessary, use gluten-free breadcrumbs)*
- 1/4 cup of red onion, chopped finely
- two minced garlic cloves
- One teaspoon of cumin powder
- One tsp of paprika
- To taste, add salt and pepper.
- One tablespoon of cooking olive oil

For Serving:
- Buns with sliders
- Lettuce stems
- cut tomatoes
- slices of avocado
- Your go-to condiments *(ketchup, mustard, mayonnaise, etc.)*

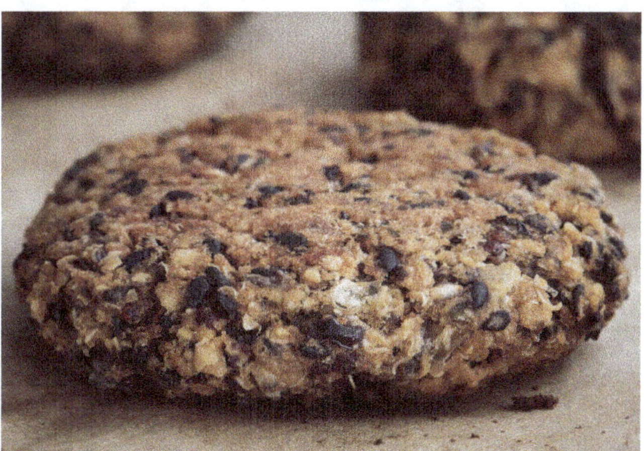

Guidelines:

Cook the quinoa according to package directions. Let it cool.

Use a fork or potato masher to mash the black beans in a large basin. For texture, leave some pieces in.

To the mashed black beans, add the cooked quinoa, breadcrumbs, red onion, chopped garlic, cumin, paprika, salt and pepper. Until all components are mixed thoroughly.

Make sure the mixture holds together properly by dividing it into tiny parts and shaping them into slider-sized patties.

In a pan over medium heat, warm the olive oil. The sliders should be cooked through and golden brown after 3 to 4 minutes on each side.

If preferred, toast the slider buns. Put a slider patty on each bun's lower half. Add slices of avocado, tomatoes and lettuce on top.

Place your preferred condiments on the upper portion of the bread.
If necessary, fasten the sliders with toothpicks and proceed to serve right away.

Avocado and Edamame Dip

Ingredients

- One cup of cooked and cooled shelled edamame
- 2 mature avocados, seeded and unseeded
- 1 minced garlic clove
- 2 tsp freshly squeezed lime juice
- Two tsp olive oil
- 1/4 cup finely chopped fresh cilantro
- To taste, add salt and pepper.
- *Optional:* flakes of red pepper for a little heat

Follow the directions on the box for cooking the shelled edamame. When cooked, remove the drain and let it come to room temperature.

Place the ripe avocados, fresh lime juice, olive oil, minced garlic and chilled edamame in a food processor.
Until the mixture is smooth, blend it. It may be necessary to pause and thoroughly scrape down the food processor's sides to make sure everything is fully mixed.

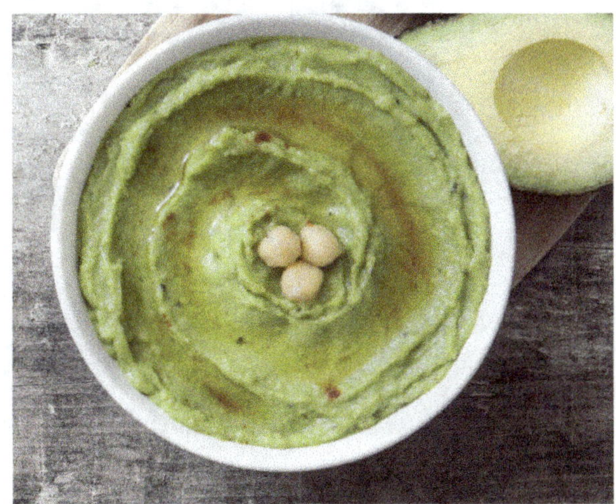

To taste, add salt and pepper.

Remember to sample the dip and adjust the spice based on your findings. Additionally, you may add red pepper flakes if you want a little spice.

Fold in the chopped cilantro after adding it to the dip. This gives the combination a splash of colour and freshness.

To serve, move the dip into a bowl. If you'd like, you may top it with some more cilantro and a drizzle of olive oil.

Accompany the Avocado and Edamame Dip with pita bread, sliced veggies, tortilla chips, or your preferred crackers.

Edamame and avocados in this dip provide a tonne of nutrients in addition to its delicious taste. It's ideal for get-togethers, parties and as a nutritious snack. Adapt the seasonings and amount to your own taste.

Roasted Chickpeas with Herbs

Ingredients

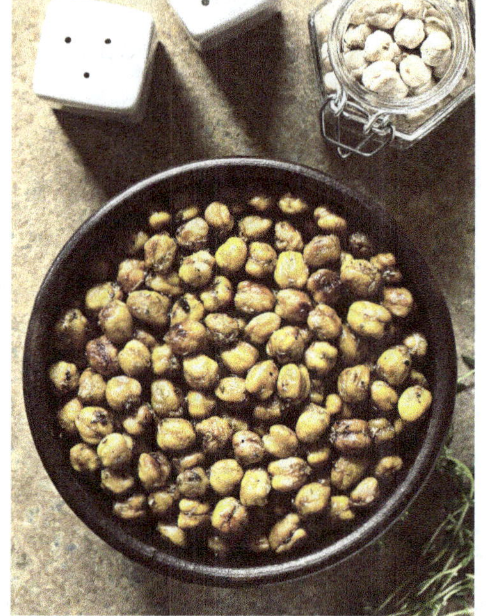

- Two cans *(15 ounces each)* of washed and drained Garbanzo beans or Chickpeas
- 2 tsp olive oil
- 1 tsp powdered garlic
- One tsp powdered onion
- A single tsp of dried thyme
- One tsp of dehydrated rosemary
- One tsp of paprika
- Half a teaspoon of cumin
- To taste, add salt and black pepper.

Guidelines:

Set the oven's temperature to 400°F, or 200°C.

Use a paper towel to pat the chickpeas dry after draining and washing them. During roasting, they will become crispier the dryer they are.

Combine the olive oil, cumin, dried thyme, dried rosemary, garlic powder, onion powder, paprika, salt and black pepper in a bowl. Taste and adjust the seasoning.

Toss in the dry chickpeas with the spice mixture, making sure they are well covered.

Arrange the seasoned chickpeas on a baking sheet in a single layer. To guarantee consistent roasting, make sure they are not packed.

After preheating the oven, put the baking sheet inside and roast the chickpeas for 25 to 30 minutes or until they are crispy and golden brown.

For uniform crispiness, stir the chickpeas or shake the pan halfway through the roasting process.

Before serving, let the roasted chickpeas cool a little. You may eat them hot or at room temperature.

Optional Additions: Use your imagination and feel free to add more spices or herbs to suit your palate. After roasting, some individuals prefer to drizzle some grated Parmesan cheese or squeeze some lemon juice over their food.

Herbed roasted chickpeas are a great snack that can be eaten on its own, mixed into salads or added crunch to soups. Try a variety of herbs and spices to discover your go-to flavour combo.

Zucchini Fritters with Tzatziki Sauce

Ingredients

Zucchini Fritters:
- Grated two medium-sized zucchini
- One tsp salt
- 1/4 cup of flour for all purposes
- 1/4 cup of Parmesan cheese, grated
- 1/4 cup of freshly chopped parsley
- two minced garlic cloves
- One huge egg that has been beaten
- To taste, add salt and pepper.
- For frying, use olive oil

Using a box grater, finely shred the zucchini. To let excess moisture drain, place the shredded zucchini in a strainer, sprinkle with salt and let set for approximately 10 minutes.

After 10 minutes, use a fresh kitchen towel to wring out the extra moisture from the shredded zucchini.

Grated zucchini, flour, Parmesan cheese, minced garlic, chopped parsley, beaten egg, salt and pepper should all be combined in a big basin.
Until all components are mixed thoroughly, stir.

In a pan over medium heat, warm the olive oil. Using a spatula to gently flatten the zucchini mixture, spoon parts onto the heated skillet.

Cook for 3–4 minutes on each side or until golden brown on both sides.

To drain any extra oil, place the fried fritters on a platter covered with paper towels.

For the Tzatziki Sauce:

- One cup of Greek yoghurt
- Half a cucumber, chopped finely, skinned, and seeded
- one minced garlic clove
- One tablespoon of freshly chopped dill
- One tablespoon of extra virgin olive oil
- one tsp lemon juice
- To taste, add salt and pepper.

Finely dice the cucumber after peeling and seeding it.

Greek yoghurt, sliced cucumber, minced garlic, chopped dill, olive oil, lemon juice, salt and pepper should all be combined in a bowl.

Until all components are properly combined, thoroughly mix.

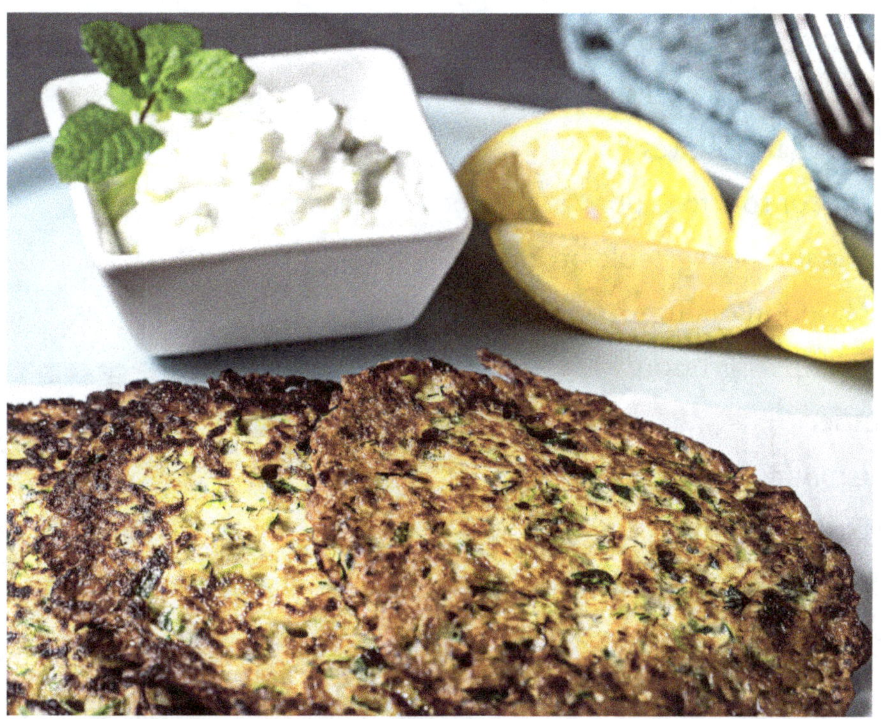

To enable the flavours to mingle, put the tzatziki sauce in the refrigerator for at least half an hour before serving.

Present the zucchini fritters warm, with a dollop of tzatziki sauce either beside or on top. Savour the savoury and delectable zucchini fritters paired with tzatziki sauce.

SOUPS AND SALADS

Lentil and Vegetable Soup

Ingredients

- One cup of washed and drained dry lentils, *either brown or green*
- 1 finely chopped onion and two diced carrots
- 2 chopped celery stalks
- 3 minced garlic cloves
- One can, or fourteen ounces chopped tomatoes
- 6 cups water or vegetable broth
- One teaspoon of cumin powder
- One tsp finely ground coriander
- One tsp of paprika
- One bay leaf
- To taste, add salt and pepper.
- Two tsp olive oil
- For garnish, use fresh cilantro or parsley *(optional)*.

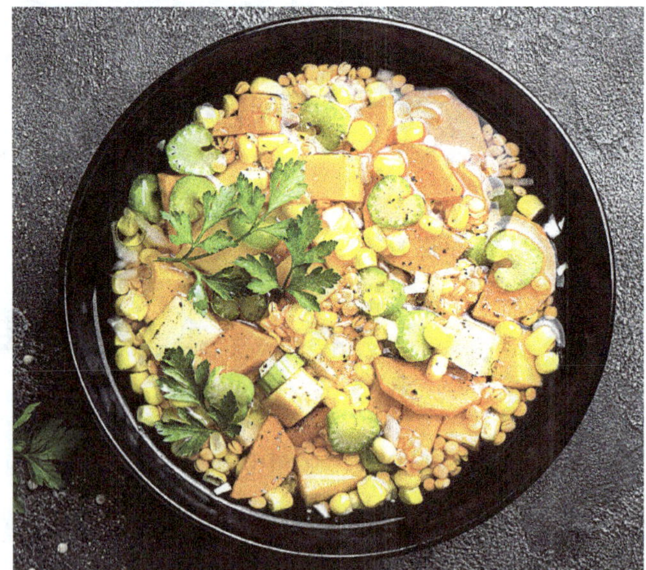

Guidelines:

Heat the olive oil in a big saucepan over medium heat.

Add the minced garlic, celery, carrots and onion. Sauté the veggies for five to seven minutes or until they are tender.

Combine the paprika, coriander and ground cumin with the veggies. To thoroughly mix in the spices, toss the veggies.

After adding the diced tomatoes, simmer for a further five minutes to let the flavours combine.

To the saucepan, add the bay leaf, rinsed lentils and vegetable broth *(or water)*. After bringing the soup to a boil, lower the heat to a simmer, cover it and let it cook for 25 to 30 minutes or until the lentils are soft.

Add salt and pepper to taste while preparing the soup. *As necessary,* adjust the seasoning.

Take out the bay leaf and throw it away.

If preferred, top the hot lentil and vegetable soup with chopped cilantro or fresh parsley.

Feel free to add potatoes, spinach or kale to this basic recipe to make it your own.

Grilled Portobello Mushroom Salad

Ingredients

- 4 big Portobello mushrooms with their stems trimmed for the salad
- Two tsp olive oil
- To taste, Salt and pepper.
- 8 cups of mixed salad greens—spinach, rocket or any other green you like.
- Half a cup of cherry tomatoes

- One cucumber and two finely sliced red onions
- 1/4 cup of crumbled feta cheese *(optional)*
- 1/4 cup finely chopped fresh parsley *(for garnish)*

For the Dressing:

- Balsamic vinegar
- 1/4 cup Turmeric
- 3 tablespoons of extra virgin
- One tsp Dijon mustard
- 1 minced garlic clove
- To taste, Salt and pepper.

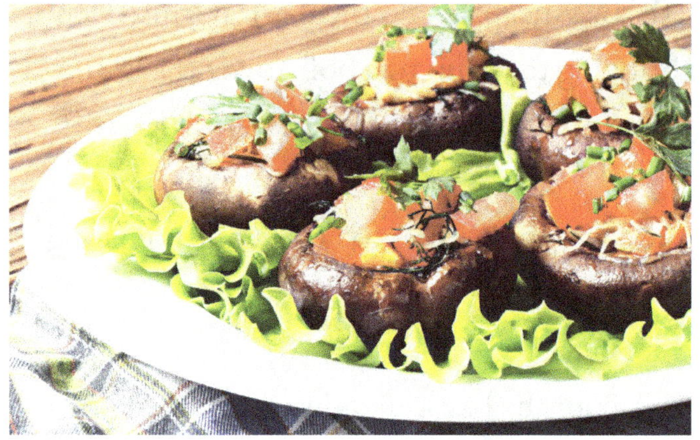

Guidelines:

Set the temperature of your grill pan or grill to medium-high.

Add salt and pepper to the portobello mushrooms after brushing them with olive oil. The mushrooms should be cooked and have grill marks after around 4–5 minutes on each side of the grill.

Before slicing them into strips, take them from the grill and allow them to cool.

Mix the red onion, cucumber, cherry tomatoes and mixed greens in a big salad dish.

Prepare the Dressing:
Combine the extra virgin olive oil, Dijon mustard, minced garlic, balsamic vinegar, salt and pepper in a small bowl and whisk until thoroughly blended.

Combine the salad with the grilled slices of portobello mushrooms and over the salad, drizzle with the dressing and toss lightly to mix.

Add some crumbled feta cheese on top *if you'd like*. Add fresh parsley as a garnish.

Serve the salad with grilled portobello mushrooms as a side dish or as a main course right away.

This salad is tasty and adaptable at the same time. Feel free to add grilled chicken for added protein or your favourite veggies to make it your own.

Chickpea and Kale Caesar Salad

Ingredients

Regarding the Salad:
- One bunch of cleaned and sliced kale
- One can (15 oz) of rinsed and drained chickpeas
- 1/2 a cup of cherry tomatoes
- Grated Parmesan cheese, 1/2 a cup

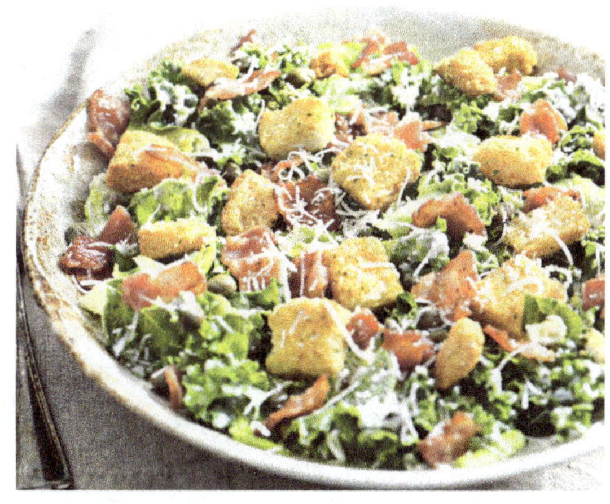

For the Caesar Dressing:
- one-half cup mayonnaise
- 2 tsp Dijon mustard
- two minced garlic cloves
- Two minced anchovy fillets *(optional)*
- 1 spoonful of sauce from Worcestershire
- One tablespoon of lemon juice
- 1/4 cup of Parmesan cheese, grated

- To taste, Salt and pepper.

For the optional croutons:
- 2 cups of day-old bread, cubed
- Two tsp olive oil
- 1 tsp powdered garlic
- To taste, Salt and pepper.

Guidelines:

Mix mayonnaise, Dijon mustard, chopped garlic, Worcestershire sauce, grated Parmesan cheese, lemon juice, salt and pepper in a bowl.

If using anchovies, stir them in as well. Taste and adjust the seasoning.

Turn the oven on to 375°F, or 190°C.

Mix the bread cubes with salt, pepper, garlic powder and olive oil.

On a baking sheet, spread out the cubes and bake for ten to fifteen minutes or until golden and crispy.

Chop the kale, add the chickpeas, cherry tomatoes and grated Parmesan cheese to a large mixing bowl.

When the salad is well covered, add the Caesar dressing and toss again.

Spoon the salad onto bowls or plates and serve right away. *If you're using croutons,* add them to the salad just before serving to keep them crunchy.

Sweet Potato and Coconut Curry Soup

Ingredients

A tasty and cosy soup, Sweet Potato and Coconut Curry Soup blends the naturally sweet taste of sweet potatoes with the rich, creamy taste of coconut milk.

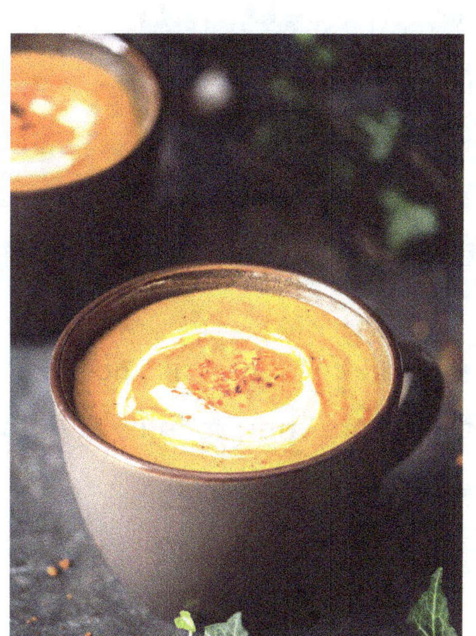

- 2 big sweet potatoes, chopped and skinned
- One 14-oz can of coconut milk
- One onion, chopped finely
- 2 minced garlic cloves
- One spoonful of curry powder
- One teaspoon of cumin powder
- One tsp finely ground coriander
- 1/2 a teaspoon of turmeric
- 1/4 tsp cayenne *(adjust according to taste)*
- 4 cups of broth made with vegetables
- To taste, Salt and pepper.
- Two teaspoons of vegetable or coconut oil
- Finely chopped fresh cilantro *(for garnish)*
- Slices of lime *(for serving)*

Guidelines:

In a large saucepan set over medium heat, warm the coconut oil. Add the minced garlic and onions and cook until they soften.

To the saucepan, add curry powder, turmeric, cayenne pepper, ground cumin and powdered coriander. Toss to evenly distribute the spices over the onions and garlic.

Sweet potatoes should be diced and added to the saucepan. Sauté for a few more minutes.

After adding the veggie broth, heat the mixture until it boils. Once the sweet potatoes are soft, reduce the heat, cover and simmer for 15 to 20 minutes.

After the sweet potatoes are cooked, purée the soup until it's smooth using an immersion blender.

You may transfer the soup to a blender in stages and puree it until smooth if you don't have an immersion blender.

Add the coconut milk and taste-test to adjust the seasoning of the soup. To give the flavours time to mingle, simmer for a further 5 to 10 minutes.

Serve the soup hot, with lime wedges and chopped cilantro on the side.

Quinoa and Roasted Vegetable Salad

Ingredients

- 1 cup of rinsed and drained quinoa
- One medium eggplant
- 1 diced zucchini
- one diced red pepper
- one chopped yellow pepper
- 1 diced red onion
- 2 cups of water or vegetable broth

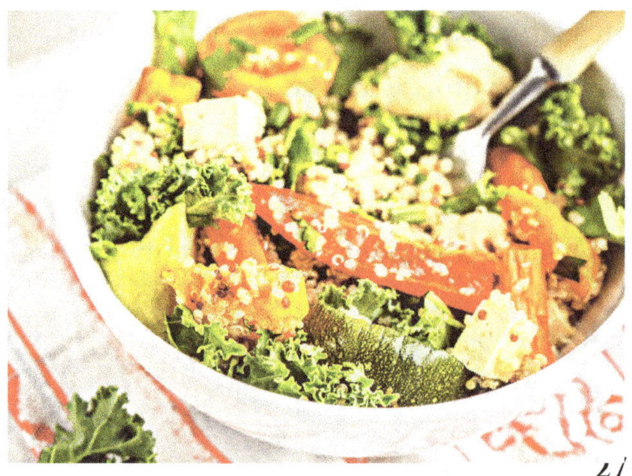

- Three teaspoons of olive oil
- To taste, Salt and pepper.
- One tsp of dehydrated oregano
- A single tsp of dried thyme
- Half a cup of cherry tomatoes
- 1/4 cup of crumbled feta cheese *(optional)*
- Finely chopped fresh cilantro or parsley for garnish

Regarding the Dressing:
- 3 teaspoons of olive oil
- Half a tsp balsamic vinegar
- 1 minced garlic clove
- To taste, Salt and pepper.

Guidelines:

Set oven temperature to 400°F, or 200°C.

Quinoa should be combined with water or vegetable broth in a medium pot. After bringing to a boil, lower the heat to a simmer, cover and let the quinoa cook for about 15 minutes or until the liquid has been absorbed.

Using a fork, fluff and put aside.

Diced eggplant, zucchini, red pepper, yellow pepper and red onion should all be combined in a big mixing basin.

Season with salt, pepper, dried oregano and dried thyme, then drizzle with olive oil. Vegetables should be tossed until covered evenly.

Arrange the veggies on a baking pan so they are in a single layer. Roast, tossing occasionally, in the preheated oven for 25 to 30 minutes or until the veggies are soft and beginning to brown.

In a separate bowl, mix together olive oil, balsamic vinegar, minced garlic, salt and pepper to make the dressing while the veggies are roasting.

The cooked quinoa, roasted veggies, cherry tomatoes and, *if used*, crumbled feta cheese should all be combined in a large serving dish. Over the salad, drizzle with the dressing and toss lightly to mix.

Before serving, garnish with chopped fresh cilantro or parsley.

Serve this warm or cold Quinoa and Roasted Vegetable Salad, which is not only tasty but also a fantastic source of nutrients.

MAIN COURSES – VEGETARIAN DELIGHTS

Eggplant Parmesan

Ingredients

- 1/2 an aubergine each, cut into rounds of half an inch
- Salt
- 2 cups of all-purpose flour
- 4 big, beaten eggs
- Two cups of breadcrumbs *(Italian seasoned preferred)*
- Grated Parmesan cheese, 1 cup
- Two cups of homemade or store-bought marinara sauce
- Two cups of mozzarella cheese, shredded
- Garnish with fresh basil leaves *(optional)*.

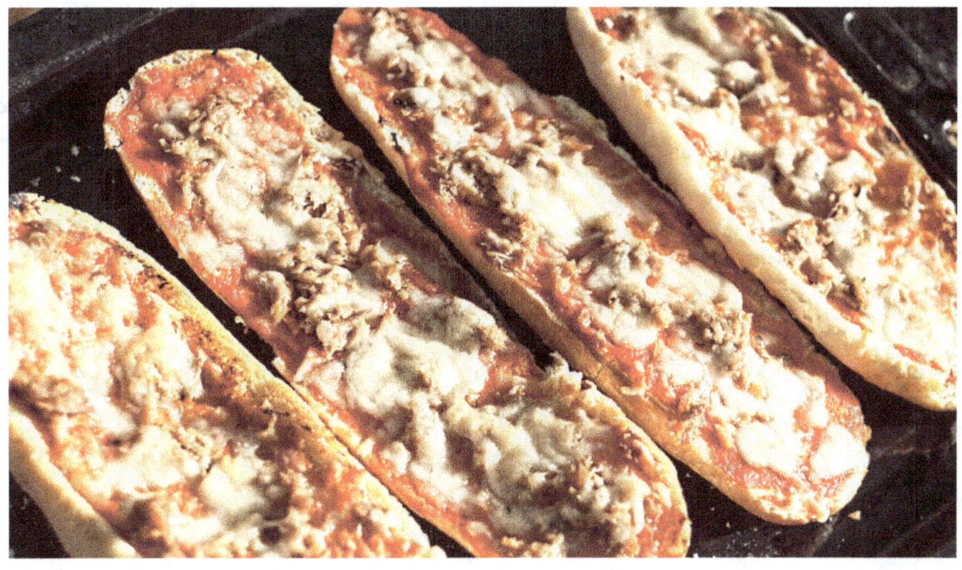

Guidelines:

Turn the oven on to 375°F, or 190°C.

After dusting the eggplant slices with salt, let them rest for approximately half an hour. This aids in removing extra moisture.

Slices of eggplant should be rinsed under cold water and dried with paper towels after 30 minutes.

Set up three small dishes at a breading station. Spoon flour into one dish; whip eggs into another; then fill the third with a breadcrumb and Parmesan cheese combination.

Shake off excess flour from each eggplant slice before dipping it in the beaten eggs, breadcrumb-Parmesan mixture and lastly pressing the breadcrumbs onto the eggplant to stick.

After lining a baking sheet with parchment paper, place the breaded aubergine slices in the preheated oven and bake for 20 to 25 minutes or until they are crisp and golden brown. Halfway through the baking time, turn the slices over.

Apply a thin layer of marinara sauce to a baking dish. Arrange the cooked eggplant slices in a layer on top, then add a layer of shredded mozzarella.

Continue layering the ingredients until all of them are utilised and then top with a layer of mozzarella.

Bake for a further 25 to 30 minutes or until the cheese is bubbling and melted.

Before serving, take it out of the oven and give it some time to rest.

If desired, garnish with fresh basil leaves.

Spaghetti Squash Primavera

Ingredients

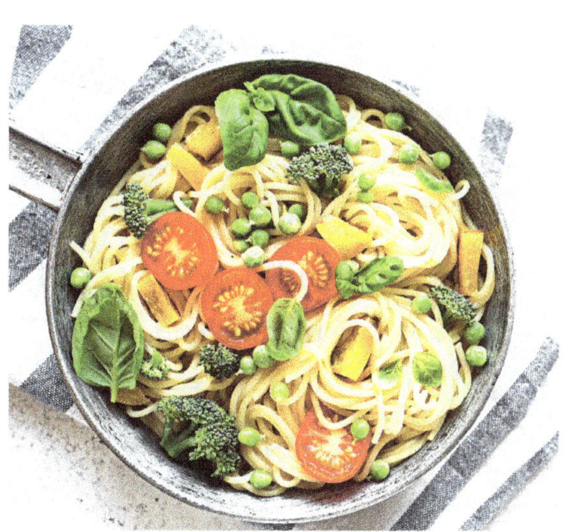

- One spaghetti squash of moderate size
- 2 tsp olive oil
- 3 minced garlic cloves
- One little red onion, cut thinly
- One red bell pepper, cut thinly
- One yellow bell pepper, cut thinly
- One finely sliced zucchini
- Half a cup of cherry tomatoes
- To taste, Salt and pepper.
- One-half tsp dried oregano
- 1/2 a teaspoon of dried basil
- 1/4 tsp optional red pepper flakes
- *For serving*, grated Parmesan cheese *(optional)*
- Use parsley or fresh basil as a garnish.

Guidelines:

Turn the oven on to 375°F, or 190°C.

Segment the spaghetti squash lengthwise in half. Using a spoon, remove the pulp and seeds.

Spoon the cut side of the squash halves onto a parchment paper-lined baking sheet. Bake for 40 to 45 minutes or until the squash is soft and readily scraped with a fork, in a preheated oven.

Heat the olive oil in a big pan over medium heat while the spaghetti squash bakes.

Garlic powder should be added and sautéed for one minute or until aromatic. Sliced red onion, yellow bell pepper, red onion and zucchini should all be added to the skillet. Cook the veggies for five to seven minutes or until they are crisp-tender.

Add the cherry tomatoes and simmer, stirring, for a further two to three minutes or until the tomatoes are cooked through.

Add salt, pepper, dried oregano, dried basil and red pepper flakes *(if using)* to the veggies to season them. Blend well.

After the spaghetti squash has finished baking, scrape the meat into strands with a fork.

Combine the sautéed veggies in a pan with the spaghetti squash strands. Mix everything together until thoroughly hot and properly mixed.

Taste and adjust the seasoning and then arrange the spaghetti squash primavera into bowls, topping it with grated Parmesan cheese and fresh basil or parsley, *if preferred*.

Mushroom and Spinach Stuffed Bell Peppers

Ingredients

- 4 big bell peppers, any hue
- One tablespoon of olive oil
- One onion, chopped finely

- Two minced garlic cloves, roughly 8 ounces (225g) chopped mushrooms, finely
- 2 cups finely chopped fresh spinach
- One cup of cooked rice or quinoa
- One cup of finely shredded mozzarella cheese *(or any other kind of cheese)*
- To taste, Salt and pepper.
- One tsp of dehydrated oregano
- One tsp of dried basil
- Half a teaspoon of optional red pepper flakes
- One 14-oz can of chopped, drained tomatoes
- *For garnish*, use fresh parsley *(optional)*.

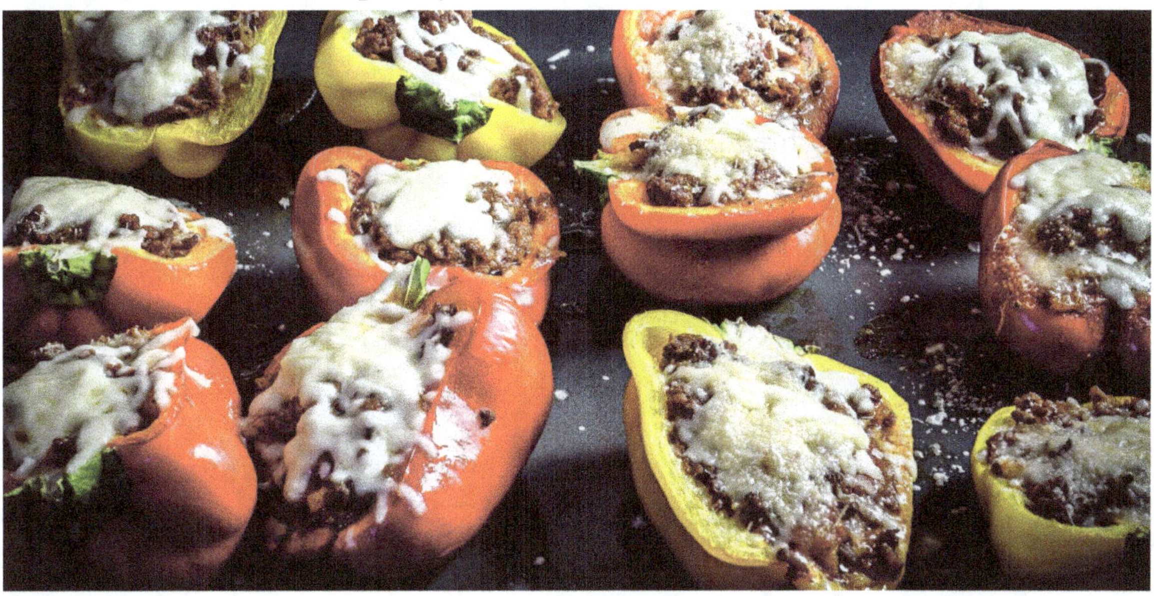

Guidelines:

Turn the oven on to 375°F, or 190°C.

Slice off the bell peppers' tops, then take out the seeds and membranes. In order to stabilise the peppers and make them stand erect, you may cut a tiny slice off the bottom.

Heat the olive oil in a big skillet over medium heat. Add the minced garlic and onions and cook until they soften.

When the mushrooms have released their moisture and become golden brown, add them to the skillet and cut them up.

Add the chopped spinach and heat, stirring, until it wilts then add salt, pepper, basil, oregano and red pepper flakes *(if using)* for seasoning.

Take the pan off of the burner and mix in the chopped tomatoes, half of the shredded cheese and cooked rice or quinoa.

Gently stuff the combination of spinach and mushrooms into each bell pepper and place the remaining shredded cheese on top of each filled pepper.

The filled peppers should be put on a roasting tray. Pour a little amount of water into the dish's bottom to keep it from sticking and to provide moisture when baking.

When the oven is hot, cover the dish with aluminium foil and bake for 25 to 30 minutes or until the peppers are soft.

After taking off the foil, bake for a further five to ten minutes or until the cheese is bubbling and melted.

If preferred, garnish the filled peppers with fresh parsley and serve them hot.

Depending on your taste, you may alter the recipe by adding other veggies, herbs or spices.

Butternut Squash and Sage Risotto

Ingredients

Risotto with butternut squash and sage is a delectable and cosy dinner.

- 1 butternut squash, chopped into little pieces after being skinned and seeded
- 2 cups Arborio rice
- One onion, chopped finely
- 4 minced garlic cloves
- half a cup of dry white wine
- Six cups of heated vegetable or chicken broth
- 1/2 a cup of grated Parmesan cheese
- Two teaspoons of freshly chopped sage
- 2 tsp butter
- Two tsp olive oil
- To taste, Salt and pepper.

Guidelines:

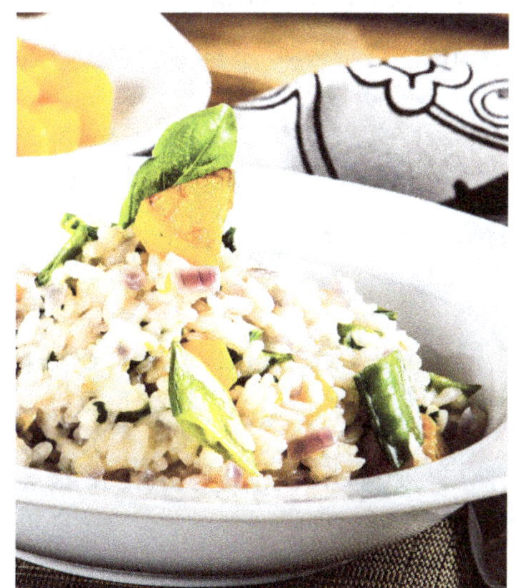

Set oven temperature to 400°F, or 200°C.

Mix the chopped butternut squash with salt, pepper and olive oil.

Roast the squash for 20 to 25 minutes or until it is soft, after spreading it out in a single layer on a baking sheet and then set aside.

Heat the olive oil and one tablespoon of butter in a big, deep skillet or saucepan over medium heat.

Add the chopped onion and simmer for three to 5 minutes or until softened.

When the garlic is aromatic, add the minced garlic and simmer for a further 1 to 2 minutes.

Once the rice is gently browned, stir in the Arborio and simmer for one to two minutes.

Till rice has absorbed most of the white wine, pour it in and stir.

One ladle at a time, slowly add the heated broth while stirring constantly.

Add the next ladle of broth when the liquid has been largely absorbed. This should be done for another 18 to 20 minutes or until the rice is creamy and cooked to al dente.

In the last five minutes of simmering, stir in the chopped sage and the roasted butternut squash pieces.

Until the rice has the right consistency, keep adding broth as required.

Take the pan off of the heat as soon as the rice is done and the risotto is creamy then add the remaining tablespoon of butter and the grated Parmesan cheese - stir.

To taste, add salt and pepper for seasoning.

Place a spoonful of the risotto into dishes or plates, *If preferred*, garnish with more parmesan and sage leaves.

Vegetable Stir-Fry with Tofu

Ingredients

- 1 solid block of diced and pressed tofu
- Two tsp soy sauce
- One tablespoon of sesame oil
- One tablespoon of vegetable oil
- 2 minced garlic cloves
- One bell pepper *(any colour)*
- 1 onion -chopped
- sliced 2 carrots
- 1 tablespoon of ginger *(powder or grated)*
- One chopped zucchini and one cup of broccoli florets
- One cup of cleaned snap peas
- 1 cup of sliced mushrooms
- 2 teaspoons of hoisin sauce
- One-tspn rice vinegar
- To taste, Salt and pepper.
- Add a garnish of sesame seeds *(optional)*.
- Chopped green onions for garnish *(optional)*
- Ready-to-serve cooked rice or noodles

Guidelines:

Tofu should be pressed to eliminate extra water and then cut into cubes.

Tofu cubes should be combined with soy sauce in a basin and let marinade for at least 15 to 20 minutes.

In a large skillet or wok, heat the vegetable oil over medium-high heat.

When the tofu cubes are added, marinade them and fry them till golden brown all over. Take out the tofu and put it aside.

If necessary, add a little more oil to the same pan. Fry the ginger and garlic until aromatic.

Add the bell pepper, onion, snap peas, broccoli, zucchini and carrots. The veggies should be stir-fried for a few minutes to make them crisp-tender.

Reintroduce the cooked tofu and veggies to the pan.

Combine rice vinegar, hoisin sauce and sesame oil in a small bowl. Drizzle the tofu and veggies with this sauce and mix everything until well combined.

To taste, add salt and pepper for seasoning. *If necessary*, adjust the flavour or sauce.

If desired, garnish with chopped green onions and sesame seeds.
Serve the tofu-and-vegetable stir-fry over cooked noodles or rice.

Add or remove veggies from this stir-fried tofu vegetable dish based on your own preferences.

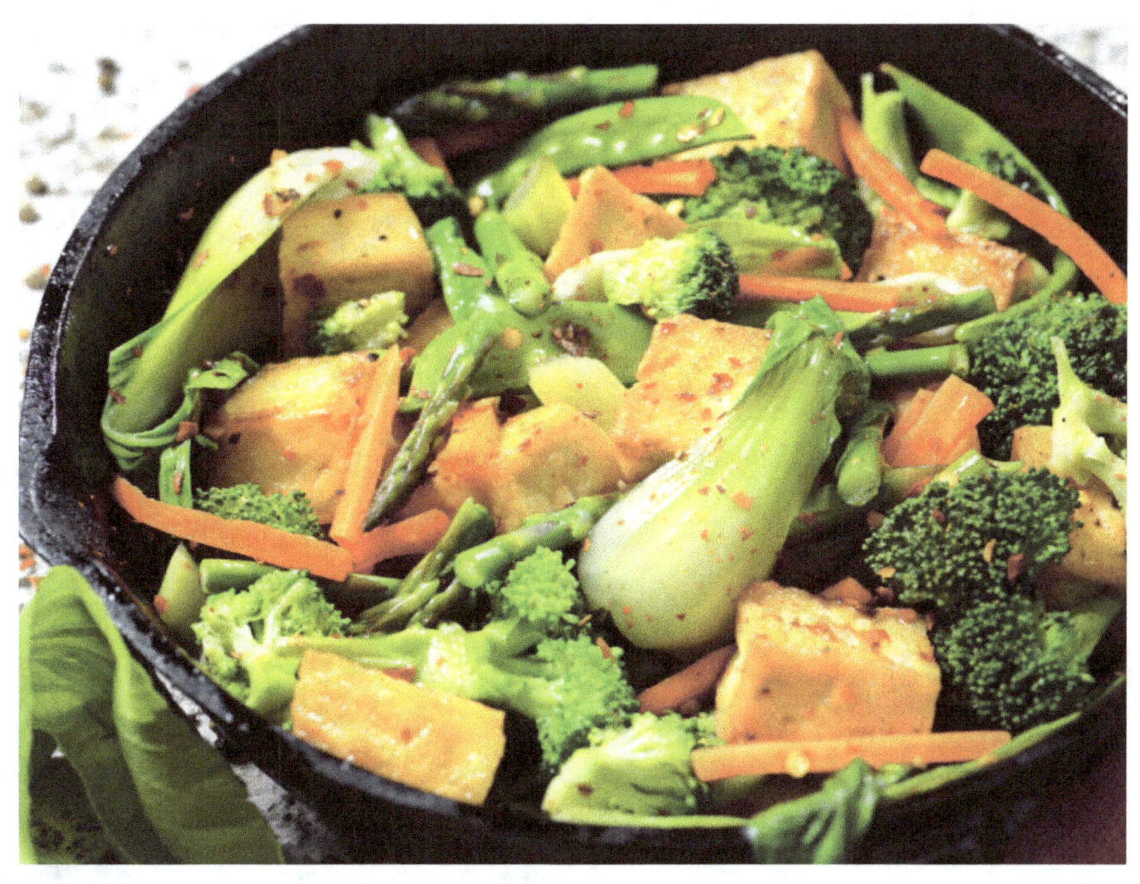

PROTEIN-PACKED MAIN COURSES

Grilled Lemon Herb Chicken

Ingredients

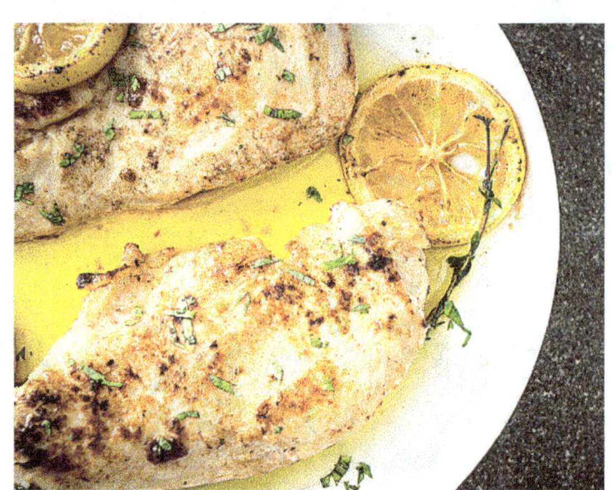

- Four skinless and boneless chicken breasts
- 1/4 cup olive oil
- 2 tsp freshly squeezed lemon juice
- 2 minced garlic cloves
- One tsp of dehydrated oregano
- A single tsp of dried thyme
- One tsp of dehydrated rosemary
- One tsp of paprika
- To taste, Salt and black pepper.
- Chopped fresh parsley *(for garnish)*
- slices of lemon *(for serving)*

Guidelines:

To make the marinade, combine the olive oil, lemon juice, minced garlic, paprika, rosemary, thyme and salt with black pepper.
Put the chicken breasts in a shallow dish or resealable plastic bag.

Ensure that every piece of chicken is well covered by pouring the marinade over it.

To marinate, close the bag or cover the dish and place it in the refrigerator for at least half an hour - *you may marinade it for many hours or even overnight to improve the flavour.*

Set your grill's temperature to medium-high.
Take the chicken out of the marinade and let the extra to fall off.

Once the grill is ready, place the chicken breasts on it and cook for 6 to 8 minutes on each side or until the chicken is no longer pink in the centre and the internal temperature reaches 165°F (74°C).

After it's done, take the chicken from the grill and give it some time to rest.

For added taste, garnish with finely chopped fresh parsley and serve with lemon wedges on the side.

Savour your Grilled Lemon Herb Chicken with salad, rice or roasted veggies, also any other favourite side dish.

This recipe yields a flavorful and juicy grilled chicken by perfectly balancing citrus and herb flavours.

Black Bean and Quinoa Burgers

Ingredients

Vegetarian or vegan burgers made with black beans and quinoa are a tasty and healthy substitute for regular meat burgers.

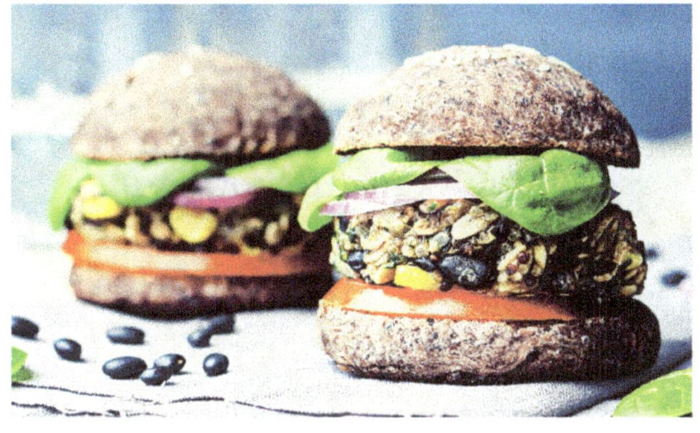

- One cup of cooked quinoa
- One can (15 oz) of rinsed and drained black beans
- 1/2 cup of red onion, chopped finely

- Half a cup of breadcrumbs *(gluten-free or whole-wheat)*
- 2 minced garlic cloves
- One teaspoon of cumin powder
- One tsp of chilli powder
- Half a teaspoon of paprika
- To taste, add salt and pepper.
- 1/4 cup tamari or soy sauce *(for a gluten-free alternative)*
- One tablespoon of extra virgin olive oil for cooking
- Whole grain buns, lettuce, tomato, avocado, onion, salsa and other toppings *are optional.*

Guidelines:

Turn the oven on to 375°F, or 190°C.

Using a fork or potato masher, roughly mash the black beans in a large basin, leaving some lumps for texture.

Add the cooked quinoa, olive oil, soy sauce, finely chopped red onion, breadcrumbs, minced garlic, ground cumin, chilli powder and paprika to the mashed black beans.

Until the ingredients are uniformly blended, thoroughly mix everything.

Create patties out of the mixture. Depending on what you choose, the size might change.

In a skillet over medium heat, preheat a little amount of olive oil. The patties should be cooked for 3–4 minutes on each side or until a golden-brown crust forms.

After transferring the patties to a parchment paper-lined baking sheet, bake them in the preheated oven for a further 15 to 20 minutes or until they are well cooked.

Top the black bean and quinoa burgers with your preferred toppings and serve them on whole grain buns. They may also be eaten over a salad without the buns.

The flavour may be improved by adding herbs, spices or even a little spicy sauce.

Salmon with Dill and Cucumber Sauce

Ingredients

Regarding the Salmon:
- 4 fillets of salmon
- To taste, Salt and pepper.
- Use olive oil for cooking.

Regarding the Cucumber and Dill Sauce:
- One cup of Greek yoghurt
- half a cucumber, chopped finely
- One tablespoon of lemon juice
- 2 teaspoons of freshly chopped dill
- To taste, Salt and pepper.

Guidelines:

Set oven temperature to 400°F, or 200°C.

On both sides, season the salmon fillets with salt and pepper. In a pan that is oven safe, warm the olive oil over medium-high heat.

With the skin side down, place the salmon fillets in the pan and sear for two to three minutes or until the skin is crispy.

After transferring the pan to the oven, warm it and bake the salmon for 10 to 12 minutes or until done to your preference.

Greek yoghurt, sliced cucumber, chopped dill and lemon juice should all be combined in a bowl for the sauce.

Thoroughly mix the ingredients until they are all equally incorporated.

Add salt and pepper to taste and season the sauce.

Take the salmon out of the oven when it's done. Spoon the cucumber and dill sauce over the salmon fillets that have been placed on plates.

If desired, garnish with more fresh dill.

Serve the salmon with your preferred side dishes, including rice, roasted potatoes or steamed veggies.

Lentil and Sweet Potato Curry

Ingredients

A tasty and nourishing recipe, lentil and sweet potato curry blends the earthy flavours of lentils and the sweetness of sweet potatoes with a dash of fragrant spices.

- 1 cup of washed and drained dried lentils *(red or green)*
- Peel and dice 2 medium-sized Sweet potatoes.
- One big onion, diced finely
- 3 minced garlic cloves
- One tablespoon of grated ginger
- One can, or 14 ounces chopped tomatoes
- One can, or 14 ounces milk from coconuts
- Curry powder
- 2 teaspoons
- One teaspoon of cumin powder
- One tsp finely ground coriander
- half a teaspoon of turmeric
- 1/4 tsp cayenne *(adjust according to taste)*
- To taste, Salt and pepper.
- 2 tsp of vegetable oil
- *To garnish*, use fresh cilantro.
- Naan bread or cooked rice ready to be served

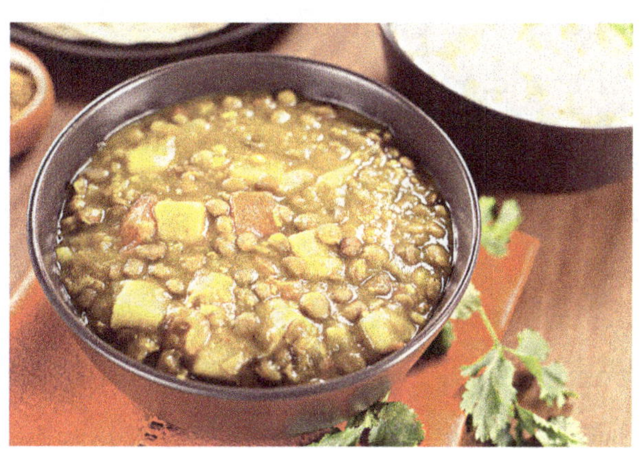

Guidelines:

Lentils should be rinsed in cold water until the water is clear.
Pour enough water into a large saucepan to cover the lentils by approximately one inch.

After bringing to a boil, lower the heat and cook the lentils until they are soft but not mushy. Remove any extra water.

Vegetable oil should be heated over medium heat in a big pan or pot then add the chopped onions and sauté.

Add the grated ginger and minced garlic and sauté for one more minute or until fragrant.

Add the turmeric, cayenne pepper, curry powder, powdered cumin, ground coriander, salt and pepper. Toasted the spices for 1 to 2 minutes.

Coat the sweet potatoes with the spice mixture by adding them chopped to the saucepan.

Include the chopped tomatoes *(with their liquids)* and the cooked lentils in the saucepan. Mix well to blend.
After adding the coconut milk and bringing the mixture to a moderate boil, lower the heat and cook the sweet potatoes until they are soft and the flavours have blended.

After tasting the curry, adjust the spices. *If desired*, add more cayenne pepper, salt or pepper.

Serve the Sweet Potato and Lentil Curry over Naan Bread or over cooked rice and add fresh cilantro as a garnish, *if preferred*.

Turkey and Veggie Skewers

Ingredients

- One pound, or around 450 grammes of cubed Turkey breast
- Cut up a variety of veggies *(such as red peppers, cherry tomatoes, zucchini, red onions and mushrooms)* into bite-sized pieces.
- Olive oil
- Juice from lemons

- Minced garlic with paprika
- Oregano, dried
- To taste, Salt and pepper.
- Metal or wood skewers; if wood, soak the skewers in water for half an hour before using.

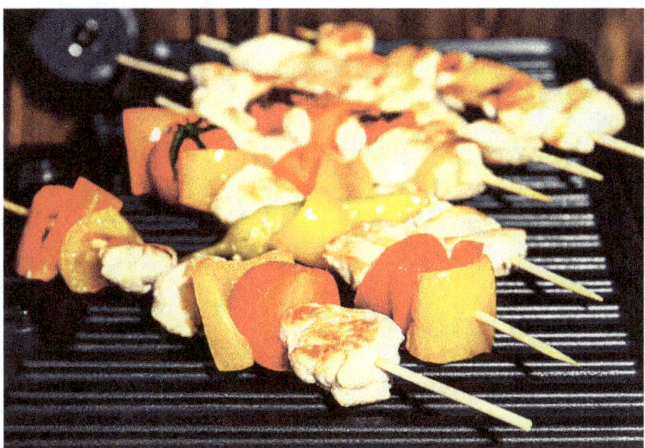

Guidelines:

Make a marinade in a bowl by combining olive oil, lemon juice, minced garlic, paprika, dried oregano, salt and pepper.

Make sure the turkey cubes are well covered by adding them to the marinade. To enable the flavours to seep in, cover the bowl and refrigerate for at least half an hour.

Finely chop the variety of veggies until the pieces are small enough to put onto skewers.

Warm up the oven or grill.

Alternating between the marinated turkey cubes and the variety of vegetables, thread them onto the skewers.

If grilling, put the skewers on a hot grill and cook, rotating regularly, for 10 to 15 minutes or until the turkey is cooked through and the veggies are soft.

Set the oven to 400°F (200°C) if you want to bake. After the vegetables are roasted and the turkey is done, place the skewers on a baking sheet and bake for about 20 to 25 minutes.

After cooking, take the skewers out of the oven or grill.
If preferred, top the heated turkey and vegetable skewers with more lemon wedges and fresh herbs.

This dish offers a tasty and nutritious choice that's ideal for a fast weekday supper or a summer BBQ.

SIDES AND ACCOMPANIMENTS

Garlic Parmesan Roasted Broccoli

Ingredients

- One pound of dried and cleaned broccoli florets
- 2 tsp olive oil
- 3 minced garlic cloves
- 1/4 cup of Parmesan cheese, grated
- To taste, Salt and pepper.
- slices of lemon, *optional for serving*

Guidelines:

Set oven temperature to 400°F, or 200°C.

Add the broccoli florets, olive oil, minced garlic, salt and pepper to a large mixing bowl. Toss to coat the broccoli with the oil and spices evenly.

Arrange the broccoli in a solitary layer onto a baking sheet that has been covered with aluminium foil or parchment paper. To guarantee consistent roasting, make sure there isn't an excessive amount of florets.

The broccoli should be roasted for 20 to 25 minutes in a preheated oven or until the edges are crispy and browned.

For even cooking, you may wish to toss the broccoli halfway during the roasting time.

When the broccoli is cooked, take it out of the oven and equally cover it with grated Parmesan cheese.

Put the baking sheet back in the oven and let it bake for a further 2 to 3 minutes or until the Parmesan has melted and become brown.

Take the Roasted Broccoli with garlic and parmesan out of the oven and place it on a platter. *If desired*, squeeze some fresh lemon juice on top.

Enjoy your flavorful Garlic Parmesan Roasted Broccoli as a nutritious snack or side dish.

You may certainly play about with the amounts of spice, Parmesan, and garlic to suit your tastes.

Quinoa and Kale Stuffed Tomatoes

Ingredients

- 6 big tomatoes
- One cup of rinsed and drained quinoa
- 2 cups chopped kale
- One little onion, diced finely

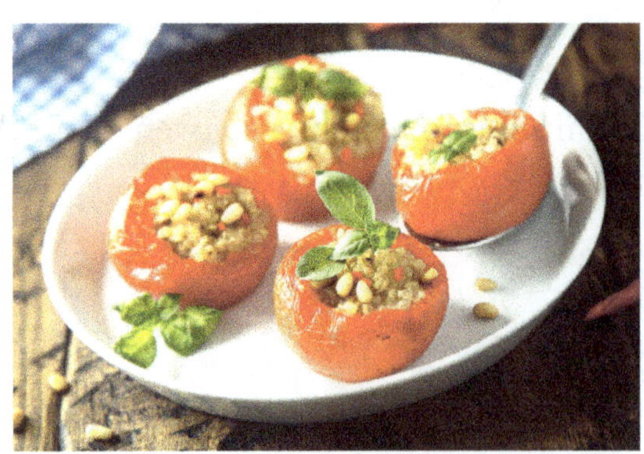

- 2 minced garlic cloves
- Half a cup of crumbled feta cheese *(optional)*
- 1/4 cup roasted pine nuts
- Two tsp olive oil
- One tsp of dehydrated oregano

- To taste, Salt and pepper.
- Use parsley or fresh basil as a garnish.

Guidelines:

Warm up the oven: Turn the oven on to 375°F, or 190°C.

To prepare the tomatoes, cut off the tops and remove the flesh and seeds, leaving the tomatoes with a hollow shell.

Season the inside with a pinch of salt and pepper and set aside.

To cook the quinoa, place it in a medium pot and add two cups of water. After bringing to a boil, lower the heat to a simmer - cover and cook the quinoa for approximately 15 minutes or until the water has been absorbed.

Using a fork, fluff the quinoa.

To sauté the veggies, use a large pan over medium heat with olive oil. Add the minced garlic and onion and cook until they become tender then add the chopped kale and cook until it wilts.

Toss the cooked quinoa, feta cheese *(if using)*, toasted pine nuts, dried oregano and sautéed veggies in a big bowl. To taste, add more salt and pepper to the seasoning.

Gently push down on the hollowed-out tomatoes as you spoon the quinoa and kale mixture inside.

Put the filled tomatoes on a baking tray and bake. Bake for 20 to 25 minutes or until the tomatoes are soft, in a preheated oven.

Before serving, sprinkle some fresh parsley or basil on top. For added flavour, you may also sprinkle a little olive oil over the top.

This meal is not only aesthetically pleasing but also nutrient-dense. It's a delicious and filling way to savour the benefits of quinoa and kale.

Cauliflower Mash with Chives

Ingredients

A tasty and low-carb substitute for regular mashed potatoes is cauliflower mash with chives.

- 1 cauliflower head that has been sliced into florets
- Two minced garlic cloves
- Two tsp butter
- 1/4 cup milk or heavy cream, *adjusted for consistency*
- To taste, Salt and pepper.
- Two teaspoons of freshly cut chives

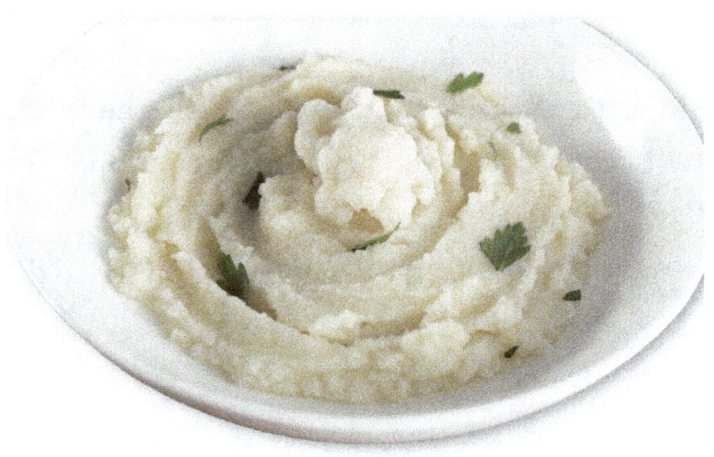

After giving the cauliflower a good rinse, cut it into florets and remove the rough stalk.

The cauliflower should be softened by steaming - *you may microwave it with a little water or use a steamer basket.*

Once the cauliflower has steamed, place it in a food processor or mash it with a potato masher until the required consistency is achieved.
Melt the butter in a pot over a medium heat. Add the minced garlic and cook, stirring for 1 to 2 minutes or until aromatic.

Cover the mashed cauliflower with the butter and garlic mixture.

To get the consistency you want, add more milk or heavy cream. Apply a little amount at first, then more as required.

To taste, add salt and pepper for seasoning and toss to blend thoroughly.

Add the chopped chives and stir. *If desired*, set aside some for garnishing.

Move the mashed cauliflower to a platter for dishing. *If desired*, garnish with more chives.

Savour the savoury flavour and creamy texture of the cauliflower mash served as a side dish with chives.

For an additional layer of flavour, you may also add shredded cheese. You can also change the consistency by adding more milk or cream.

Sauteed Green Beans with Almonds

Ingredients

- One pound of freshly cleaned and trimmed green beans
- Two tsp olive oil
- 2 minced garlic cloves
- 1/3 cup of almonds, sliced
- To taste, Salt and pepper.
- slices of lemon to serve *(optional)*

Guidelines:

Heat a big saucepan of salted water till it boils, add the green beans and simmer for 2 to 3 minutes till the green beans are brilliant green and just beginning to soften. Simmer for an extra 3 minutes to completely soften.

To halt the cooking process, drain the green beans and immediately place them in a basin of cold water.

After the green beans cool down, rinse them once more and put them aside.

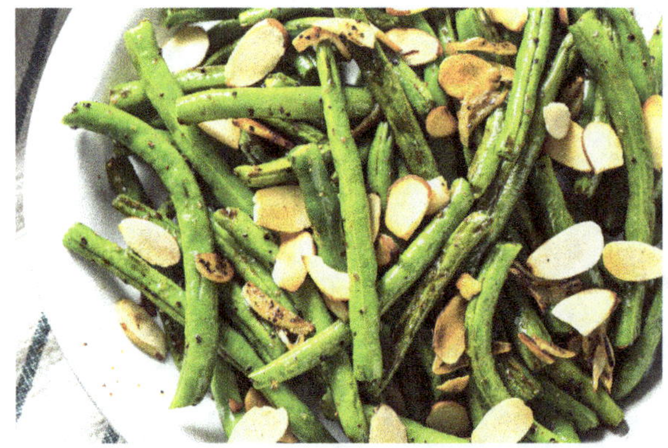

Heat the olive oil in a big skillet over medium heat and add the sliced almonds, sauté them for two to three minutes or until aromatic and golden brown.

After taking them out of the pan, set the almonds aside.

Add the minced garlic to the same pan and cook for about 1 minute or until fragrant. To the skillet, add the blanched green beans.

The green beans should be soft and crisp after 3 to 5 minutes of sautéing, stirring them often.

Reintroduce the sautéed almonds and green beans to the skillet then combine by tossing everything together.

To taste, add salt and pepper for seasoning.

Place the almonds and sautéed green beans on a platter for serving. Squeeze some fresh lemon juice on top if you want a quick hit of citrus flavour.

This dish's crunchy almonds and sautéed green beans combine to create a delicious texture and flavour that goes well as a side dish for many different kinds of dinners. To suit your tastes, add more or less lemon juice and spice.

Cilantro Lime Brown Rice

Ingredients

A tasty and wholesome side dish that goes well with many main courses, particularly Mexican or Tex-Mex cuisine, is cilantro lime brown rice.

- One cup of brown rice
- 2 cups of veggie broth or water
- 1 tablespoon of olive oil
- 2 minced garlic cloves
- One lime, both juiced and zesty

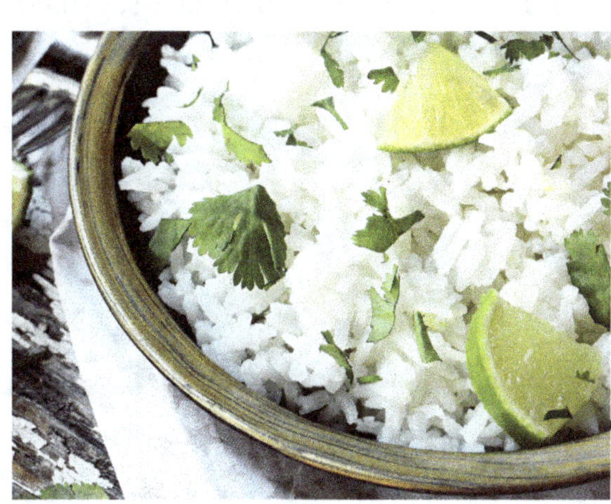

- 1/4 cup finely chopped fresh cilantro
- To taste, Salt and pepper.

Guidelines:

To get rid of extra starch, rinse the brown rice in cold water.

Place water or vegetable broth in a medium pot and add the washed brown rice to it.

After bringing to a boil, lower the heat to a simmer, cover the pot and let the rice cook for 45 to 50 minutes or until it is soft and the water has been absorbed.

As the rice cooks, prepare the flavours by heating up some olive oil in a pan over medium heat. Add the minced garlic and sauté it for one to two minutes till fragrant.
When the rice is done, move it to a big mixing basin and fluff it with a fork.

Add the chopped cilantro, lime zest, lime juice, garlic that has been sautéed, salt and pepper. Mix everything together gently until well combined.

Taste the rice and adjust the spice based on what you find to be necessary. Depending on your taste, you may add more lime juice, salt or pepper.

Accompany your preferred main course with the cilantro lime brown rice as a side dish. It pairs well with fish, tacos, grilled chicken or any other food with a Mexican flair.

For more taste and texture, you may also use other items like corn, black beans or chopped tomatoes.

DESSERTS

Chocolate Avocado Mousse

Ingredients

A delicious and healthy substitute for classic chocolate mousse is Chocolate Avocado Mousse. Avocado provides healthful lipids and adds smoothness.

- Two ripe avocados
- 1/4 cup chocolate powder, unsweetened
- 1/4 cup agave nectar or maple syrup, or to taste
- 1/4 cup almond milk *(or any other kind of milk)*
- One tsp vanilla essence
- A little amount of salt
- Whipped cream, berries, almonds or shredded coconut are *optional garnishes.*

Guidelines:

Halve the avocados and scoop out the pit. Scoop the meat into a food processor or blender and mix well.

Add the almond milk, vanilla extract, cocoa powder, maple syrup and a little amount of salt to the blender or food processor along with the avocados.

Blend the ingredients until they are creamy and smooth. To make sure everything is well mixed, scrape down the sides of the blender or food processor as necessary.

After tasting the mousse, add additional agave or maple syrup to modify the sweetness *if necessary*. If you make any changes, blend again.

Spoon the chocolate avocado mousse into glasses or bowls for serving.

To help the mousse cool and solidify, cover and chill in the refrigerator for at least 1 or 2 hours.

The chocolate avocado mousse may be served with your preferred toppings or by itself when it has cooled. Berries, almonds, shredded coconut and whipped cream are excellent choices.

This recipe is a terrific way to enjoy a creamy chocolate delight with the extra health benefits of avocados. It's also quite simple to create. You may experiment with the toppings and change the sweetness to suit your own tastes.

Berry and Almond Crisp

Ingredients

A delicious dish that combines the crispy deliciousness of an almond-flavoured topping with the sweetness of berries is called berry and almond crisp.

For the Filling:
- 4 cups of mixed berries, including strawberries, blueberries, raspberries and blackberries
- 1/2 cup of sugar, granulated
- 2 tsp cornflour
- One tablespoon of lemon juice
- One tsp vanilla essence

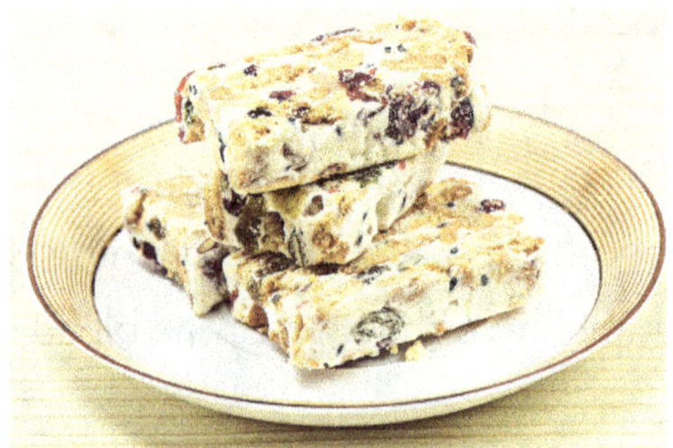

For the Topping:
- 1 cup of traditional rolled oats
- One-half cup all-purpose flour
- 1-1/2 cup almond slices
- 1/4 tsp salt and 1/2 cup packed brown sugar
- Half a cup of chilled, unsalted butter, cut into tiny cubes

Guidelines:

Set the oven temperature to 350°F (175°C). Use cooking spray or butter to grease a 9x9-inch or comparable baking dish.

The mixed berries, cornflour, lemon juice, vanilla essence and granulated sugar should all be combined in a big basin. Mix everything together until the berries are well covered.

Spread the berry mixture equally in the baking dish that has been prepared.

To make the topping, put the sliced almonds, brown sugar, rolled oats and all-purpose flour in a separate bowl. Blend well.

To the topping mixture, add the cubed, chilled butter. To make the mixture look like coarse crumbs, use your fingers or a pastry cutter to cut the butter into the dry ingredients.

Distribute the almond-oat topping equally over the baking dish's berry mixture.

Bake for 40 to 45 minutes in a preheated oven or until the berry filling is bubbling and the topping is golden brown.

Before serving, take the crisp out of the oven and let it cool for a few minutes.

Warm berry and almond crisp may be served as is, or for an added pleasure, topped with a dollop of whipped cream or a scoop of vanilla ice cream.

Greek Yogurt Parfait with Honey and Nuts

Ingredients

- One cup of plain or flavoured Greek yoghurt
- Two tsp honey or more according to taste
- 1/4 cup chopped mixed nuts, such as pistachios, walnuts or almonds
- One-fourth cup granola
- *Optional:* fresh fruits *(such kiwis, banana slices or berries).*

Guidelines:

To begin, cover the bottom of a glass or dish with a layer of Greek yoghurt.

Drizzle the yoghurt layer with one tablespoon of honey. Depending on your preferred level of sweetness, adjust the quantity of honey.

Cover the honey with a layer of chopped nuts. This gives the parfait a delicious crunch and nutty flavour.

Spread a layer of Granola over the nuts. This gives the parfait some extra texture and a healthy touch.

Continue layering on Greek yoghurt, honey, almonds and granola until the top of the glass or bowl is reached.

Optional: Garnish your parfait with fresh fruits to add more flavour and freshness, such as kiwis, banana slices or berries.

Finally, drizzle a little extra honey over the top to give it a last touch.

Take a spoon and savour this delectable Greek yoghurt parfait topped with almonds and honey.

You are welcome to alter the parfait to suit your own tastes. To make variants of this delicious dessert, try experimenting with other kinds of nuts, fruits or flavoured Greek yoghurt.

Pumpkin Protein Bars

Ingredients

- 1 cup pureed pumpkin
- Half a cup of almond butter *(or any other nut butter)*
- 1/4 cup maple syrup or honey
- two tsp of essence from vanilla
- 1 cup protein powder with vanilla extract
- One cup of rolled oats
- Half a cup of chopped nuts, such as almonds, pecans or walnuts
- Half a cup of raisins or dried cranberries
- 1 tsp finely ground cinnamon
- One-half tsp ground nutmeg
- 1/4 tsp salt

Set the oven temperature to 350°F (175°C). Line a baking dish with parchment paper or grease it.

Place pumpkin puree, almond butter, maple syrup or honey and vanilla essence in a large mixing dish. Blend until well combined.

To the wet mixture, add the protein powder, rolled oats, chopped almonds, raisins or dried cranberries, powdered nutmeg, ground cinnamon and salt and mix until well combined.

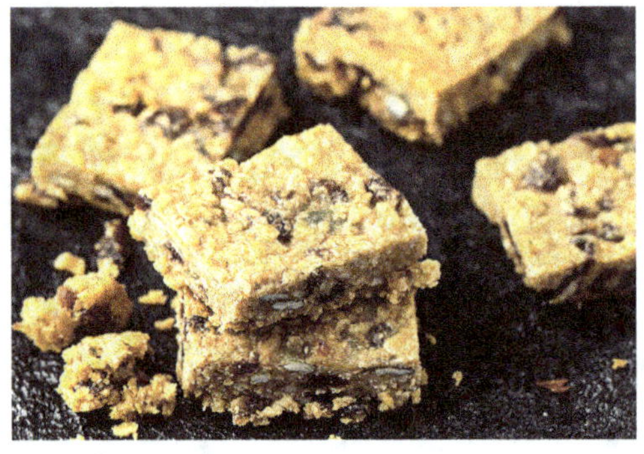

Spoon the mixture evenly onto the baking dish that has been preheated. Firmly press it down to form a tight layer.

Place the baking dish in the preheated oven and bake for approximately 20 to 25 minutes or until the sides are golden brown and a toothpick inserted into the centre comes out clean.

Let the bars cool fully in the baking dish before cutting. After they've cooled, cut them into individual bars with a sharp knife.

Optional Drizzle: You may cover the top of the bars with a thin layer of glaze or melted chocolate to add a special touch.

To maintain freshness, keep the pumpkin protein bars in the refrigerator in an airtight container. They may be packed separately for convenient grab-and-go snacks.

Coconut Chia Seed Pudding

Ingredients

Easy to prepare, Coconut Chia Seed Pudding is a tasty and nourishing dessert or brunch choice. Chia seeds are a beneficial addition to your diet since they are high in fibre, protein and omega-3 fatty acids.

- One-fourth cup chia seeds
- One cup coconut milk or *any other kind of milk you like*
- One to two teaspoons of sweetener, such agave nectar, honey or maple syrup
- Half a teaspoon of extract from vanilla
- A little amount of salt
- Fresh fruit and shredded coconut as a garnish *(optional)*

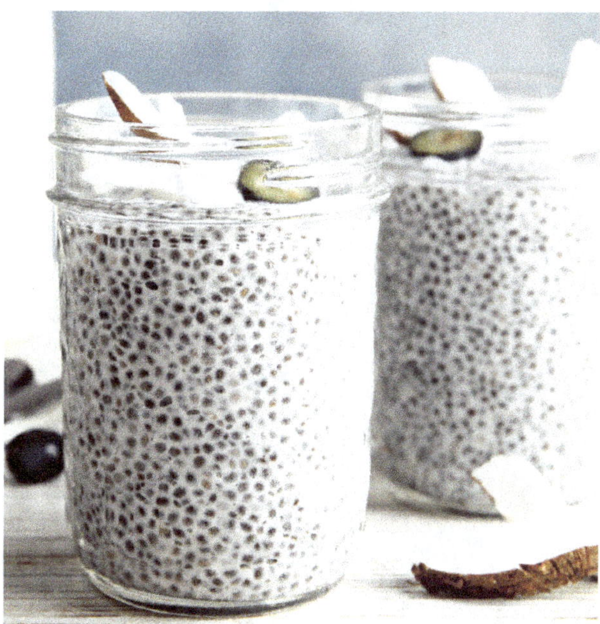

Guidelines:

Chia seeds, coconut milk, sugar, vanilla essence and a little amount of salt should all be combined in a dish.

Make sure the chia seeds are dispersed evenly by giving it a good stir.

Place a lid on the bowl and place it in the refrigerator for a minimum of four hours or overnight. The liquid will be absorbed by the chia seeds during this time, giving the mixture a pudding-like consistency.

To get a smooth texture and break up any clumps, give the custard a vigorous stir once it has set.

After tasting the custard, add additional sweetener if necessary to make it more sweet.

Present the Chia Seed Pudding with Coconut in separate dishes or jars. Add shredded coconut and fresh fruit, such as banana slices or berries, on top. Savour this nutritious and filling meal, snack or dessert—coconut chia seed pudding.

You may alter the recipe by using your preferred toppings, such as chocolate drizzle, granola or almonds. You may be creative and customise this dish to suit your own tastes with this adaptable recipe.

BEVERAGES

Green Protein Smoothie

Ingredients

- One cup of fresh spinach leaves or kale *for a more flavorful option*
- Half a cucumber, cut into slices and peel
- 1/2 an avocado
- Half a banana, for added sweetness
- 1 scoop of your preferred protein powder *(whey, hemp,or pea protein - for example)*
- One tablespoon of flax or chia seeds
- One cup almond milk or any other kind of milk you like
- Cubes of ice *(optional)*
- Maple syrup or honey *(optional; adds sweetness)*

Guidelines:

After giving the spinach *(or kale)* leaves a good wash, add them to the blender and add the almond milk, protein powder, chia seeds *(or flaxseeds)*, banana, avocado and cucumber slices.

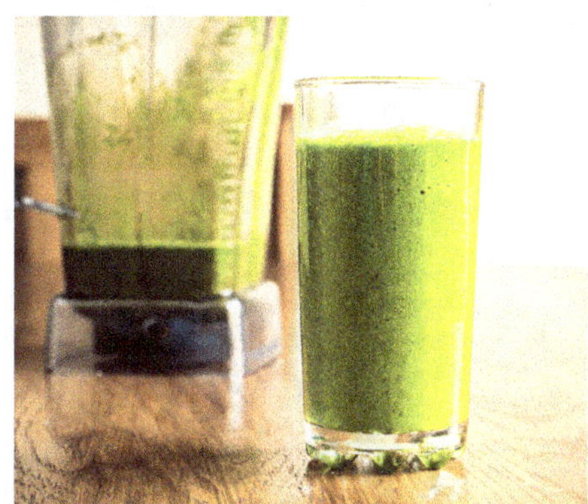

You may also add a few ice cubes if you'd like your smoothie to be cooler.

Blend every item until it becomes creamy and smooth.

After tasting the smoothie, add more honey or maple syrup to modify the sweetness *if necessary*.

Enjoy the green protein smoothie after pouring it into a glass.

For extra freshness, you may add additional ingredients like ginger, mint leaves or a little amount of lemon juice. To fit your nutritional needs, you may also use a different kind of milk or protein powder.

Berry Blast Protein Shake

Ingredients

Enjoy the benefits of berries, which are high in antioxidants, and add protein to your diet with the tasty and healthy Berry Blast Protein Shake.

- One cup of mixed berries, including blackberries, raspberries, blueberries and strawberries
- 1 scoop of the protein powder of your choice *(berry or vanilla flavoured)*
- One cup of milk, either plant-based or dairy *(such as coconut, soy or almond milk).*
- Greek yoghurt in a half-cup
- One tablespoon of *optional* chia seeds
- One tablespoon of maple syrup or honey *(optional; added for sweetness)*
- Cubes of ice *(optional)*

Guidelines:

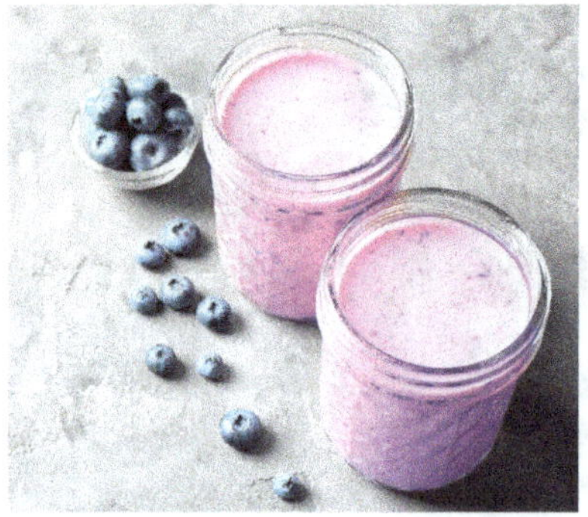

To prepare the berries, give them a thorough wash. Hull and chop any bigger berries, such as strawberries, *if using them.*

Put the mixed berries, Greek yoghurt, milk, protein powder, chia seeds *(if using)*, and sweetener *(if preferred)* in a blender.

Process the ingredients in a blender until a creamy, smooth consistency is reached. To get the right texture, you may add more milk if the shake is too thick.

Based on your taste preferences, modify the thickness or sweetness of the shake. *If necessary*, add more liquid or sweetener.

Pour the Berry Blast Protein Shake into a glass to serve. To make your drink cooler and more refreshing, feel free to add some ice cubes.

Optional Garnish: Add a sprig of mint or a few whole berries as a decorative touch.

Savour every mouth watering bite of your Berry Blast Protein Shake - It makes a nutritious snack or an excellent drink after working out.

Cucumber Mint Infused Water

Ingredients

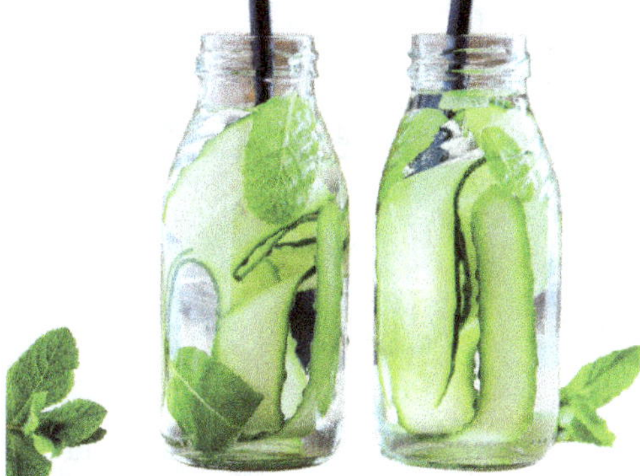

- One cucumber, cut thinly
- half a cup of fresh mint leaves
- One finely sliced lemon *(optional)*
- Cubes of ice

Instructions for Water:

Rinse the cucumber well, along with the mint leaves and lemon, *if using*.

Cut the lemon and cucumber into thin rounds. You may also gently muddle the cucumber slices to release more of their essence if you want a stronger flavour.

Fill a pitcher with the cucumber slices, mint leaves and lemon slices *(if using)*.

To further enhance the cool, refreshing taste of the infused water, add ice cubes to the pitcher.
Cover the cucumber, mint and lemon slices in the pitcher with cold water.
To disperse the flavours, carefully stir the ingredients.

To let the flavours to merge, place the infused water in the refrigerator for at least 1 or 2 hours. You may chill it overnight for a more potent infusion.

If necessary, replenish the pitcher with ice cubes before serving.

Pour the water with the cucumber-mint infusion into glasses, then enjoy the revitalising beverage.

You may play about with the amounts of lemon, mint, and cucumber to get the exact flavour profile you want. This drink has a bit of natural flavour and is delightful as well as a fantastic method to remain hydrated.

Golden Turmeric Latte

Ingredients

Due to turmeric's anti-inflammatory qualities, the Golden Turmeric Latte, also referred to as "Golden Milk," is a warm and pleasant beverage with many possible health advantages.

- One cup of milk *(dairy, almond, coconut, soy, etc.)* of your choosing

- half a teaspoon of turmeric powder
- 1/4 tsp ground cinnamon
- 1/8 tsp ground ginger
- One sprinkle of black pepper, which helps turmeric's curcumin be better absorbed.
- One teaspoon of maple syrup or honey *(adjust to taste)*
- *Optional*: One-half tsp coconut oil *(to enhance flavour)*

Guidelines:

Heat the milk in a small saucepan over medium heat. Take care not to allow it to boil.

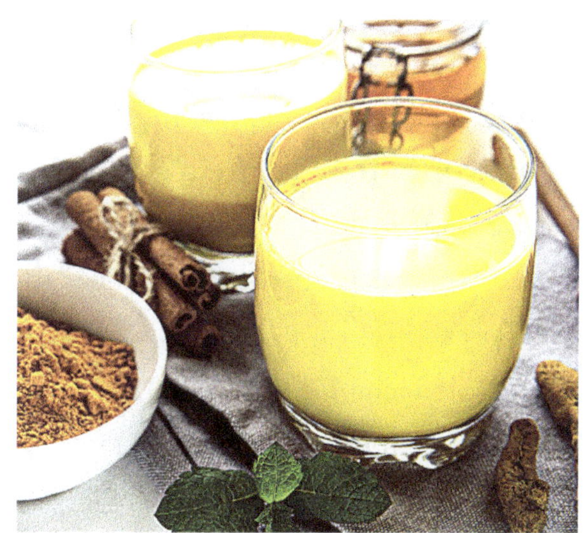

To the milk, add the ground turmeric, ginger, cinnamon and a little teaspoon of black pepper.

To make sure the spices are properly combined and to prevent lumps from developing, whisk the mixture constantly.

For extra richness, you may optionally add coconut oil. This aids in the absorption of turmeric in addition to taste.

The mixture should be heated further until it is hot but not boiling. It is important not to boil it so that the flavours may combine.

After taking the pot off the stove, taste and add honey or maple syrup to sweeten the golden turmeric latte and to suit your tastes, adjust the sweetness.

Transfer the golden turmeric latte into your preferred cup and enjoy the warming and sustaining concoction.

Spinach and Pineapple Detox Smoothie

Ingredients

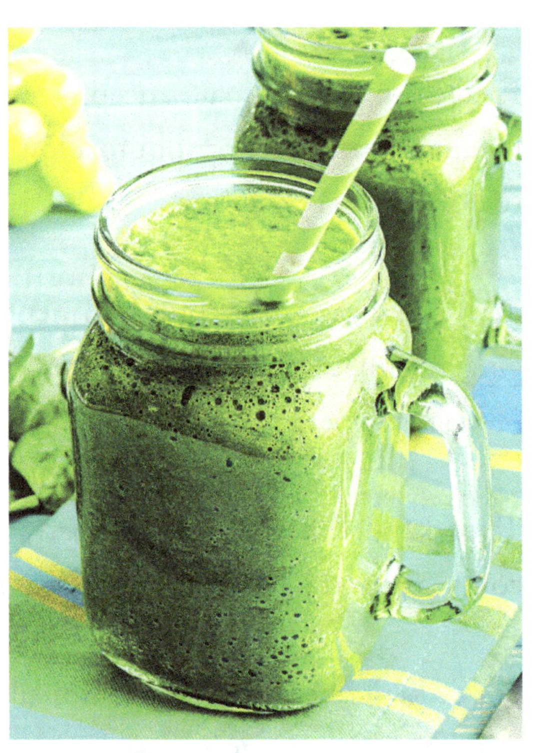

- One cup of raw spinach
- 1 cup of frozen or fresh pineapple, chopped
- Half a cucumber, cut into slices and peel
- Half a lemon, squeezed;
- half an inch of peeled and grated Ginger
- One tablespoon of *optional* chia seeds
- *To get the right consistency*, add 1 to 2 glasses of Water or Coconut water.
- Cubes of ice *(optional)*

Guidelines:

Clean the spinach leaves, chop the pineapple, peel and grate the ginger and peel and slice the cucumber.

Place the diced pineapple, sliced cucumber, grated ginger, lemon juice and chia seeds in a blender along with the fresh spinach.

Depending on the thickness or thinness of your smoothie, add one to two glasses of water or coconut water.

Process all ingredients in a blender until smooth. You may add ice cubes and mix again until they are completely blended if you would want your smoothie to be cooler.

If the smoothie is too thick, gradually add additional liquid until the right consistency is reached.

If necessary, adjust the flavours by tasting the smoothie. If you would like, you may add honey or additional lemon juice for acidity.
Immediately pour the smoothie into a glass and serve. *If desired*, you may also add a few chia seeds or more cucumber slices as a garnish.

This detox smoothie with spinach and pineapple is nutrient-rich and refreshing. Ginger offers a zest and may help with detoxification, pineapple contributes natural sweetness and vitamin C, cucumber adds moisture, and lemon juice adds a blast of citrus flavour. Spinach supplies critical vitamins and minerals. If included, the chia seeds provide fibre and omega-3 fatty acids.

TIPS FOR MEAL PLANNING AND PREPPING

Weekly Meal Planning Guide

You can eat a well-balanced diet and save time and money by organising your meals for the week. Here is a guide to assist you in organising your weekly food plan:

Step 1: Evaluate Your Calendar
Take a look at your job hours, social engagements and any other activities that can interfere with the time you have to prepare meals each week.

Step 2: Establish Objectives
Establish your dietary objectives, like maintaining a balanced diet, gaining muscle or managing your weight.

Step 3: Make a weekly menu with three courses each day.

Step 4: Create a shopping list
Enumerate every component that your meal calls for for the next week. Look through your fridge and pantry to see what you already have.

Step 5: Cooking in batches
To save time throughout the week, prepare certain items ahead of time, such as cutting vegetables or marinating meats.

Step 6: Show Flexibility

Unpredictability is a common feature of life. On hectic days, prepare easy dishes like stir-fries or simple salads as a backup.

Step 7: Management of Portion Size

To prevent overindulging, think about portion proportions. Use smaller dishes as required.

Step 8: Munchies

Make plans for wholesome snacks to keep you energised in between meals, including fruits, almonds or yoghurt.

Step 9: Drink plenty of water

Remember to drink plenty of water. Excellent options include infused water, herbal drinks and water.

Step 10: Examine and Modify

Examine what went well and what didn't at the conclusion of the week. In light of this, modify your strategy for the next week.

Recall that this is only an example guide. You are welcome to alter it to suit your tastes, dietary requirements and nutritional requirements.

Batch Cooking Tips for Busy Days

Batch cooking is an excellent time-saving tactic for stressful work days since it lets you prepare meals ahead of time. The following advice will assist you in bulk cooking:

Create Your Menu: Select dishes that are simple to double or triple and that freeze well.

- Select items that are adaptable and can be utilised to a variety of recipes.

Invest in High-Quality Containers: Make use of a range of freezer-safe containers, including freezer bags and glass and plastic containers.

- To maintain freshness, mark containers with the date and contents.

Select Recipes That Go in the Freezer:
- Pay attention to recipes like casseroles, soups, stews and sauces that freeze nicely.

- Steer clear of recipes that call for components that are difficult to freeze or reheat, such as some vegetables with a high water content *(like lettuce)*.

Basics of Batch Cooking:
- Make big quantities of basic ingredients that may be used in a variety of dishes, such as quinoa, rice or roasted vegetables.

- Cook proteins *(beans, meat and chicken)* in large quantities for a variety of recipes.

Use Your Instant Pot or Slow Cooker: These kitchen tools are great for large quantities of food. Come home to a ready-to-eat dinner by preparing the ingredients early in the day.

- Meats and stews that are slow-cooked often freeze and reheat nicely.

Plan Your Time: Designate a certain day, such as a Sunday afternoon, for cooking in bulk.

- To save time, prepare your meals, arrange the materials and expedite the cooking procedure.

Portion Control: For easier reheating, divide prepared dishes in bulk into amounts that are suitable for a person or a family.

- This reduces waste and facilitates grabbing a fast supper.

Freeze in Flat Layers: Freeze liquids, such as soups or sauces, in flat, clearly marked bags to save up freezer space. You may arrange them vertically when they're frozen.

Rotation System: To make sure you eat older frozen meals before using newer ones, use a first-in, first-out rotation.

- Check your freezer often to be informed about what's available.

Try Double Batching: When preparing regular meals, think about doubling the amount and freezing half for later use.

- In this manner, you may progressively accumulate a range of frozen meals without scheduling certain days for batch cooking.

Incorporate Breakfast and Snacks: For easy morning meals, don't forget to batch prepare foods like muffins, granola bars or breakfast burritos.

- Make wholesome grab-and-go choices like portioned almonds or chopped vegetables.

Keep a Well-Stocked Pantry: To make sure you always have alternatives, keep your pantry well-stocked with non-perishable goods to go along with your frozen dinners.

You can streamline your meal preparation, save time and make sure you always have wholesome, simple meals on hand on hectic days by putting these batch cooking methods into practice.

Proper Storage of Vegetables and Proteins

Vegetables and proteins must be stored properly to retain their nutritional content, freshness and to stop the formation of dangerous germs.

The following are broad recommendations for protein and vegetable storage:

Vegetables: Chilling
The majority of veggies should be kept refrigerated to delay ripening and avoid spoiling.

Potatoes, onions and garlic are an exception; they should be kept outside of the refrigerator in a cold, dark and dry environment.

Control of Moisture:
To keep leafy greens and herbs wet, store them in the vegetable crisper in perforated plastic bags.

To keep moisture in, store veggies like bell peppers, carrots and celery in plastic bags with a wet paper towel inside.

Keep Sensitive and Ethylene-Producing Vegetables Apart:

Certain fruits and vegetables release gas called ethylene, which may quicken the ripening of neighbouring produce that is susceptible to ethylene. Keep them apart in storage.

Producers of ethylene: Tomatoes, Bananas and Apples.
- Broccoli, carrots, and leafy greens are ethylene-sensitive.

Prevent Crowding:

For optimal air circulation, keep the refrigerator shelves from becoming too crowded.

Proteins: Cooling

To inhibit the development of germs, keep raw meat, poultry and fish in the refrigerator at or below 40°F (4°C).

Use airtight receptacles or firmly wrap proteins in foil or plastic wrap.

Separation:

Keep distinct protein types apart to avoid cross-contamination.

Raw meats should be kept on the lowest shelf to avoid leaking onto other food items.

Use-By Dates:

To guarantee freshness and safety, heed the use-by dates on proteins that are packaged.

Freezing:

- If you are not going to utilise proteins in the next several days, freeze them.

- To avoid freezer burn, place proteins in airtight containers or freezer bags.

Defrosting:

You may use the microwave, refrigerator or cold running water to thaw frozen proteins.

- To prevent the formation of germs, avoid thawing proteins at room temperature.

Prepared Proteins:

To avoid spoiling, cooked proteins should be refrigerated or frozen within two hours after cooking.

Do remember that different veggies and proteins could need different storage conditions, so it's important to take each item into account. To guarantee the quality and security of the goods you keep, always heed any special instructions on the box and pay close attention to food safety regulations.

Balancing Nutrients in Vegetarian and Protein-rich Meals

To ensure your body receives all the necessary nutrients, it is essential to balance the nutrients in vegetarian and protein-rich diets.

Plant-based protein sources like quinoa, almonds and edamame can provide a full spectrum of amino acids.

Whole grains like brown rice, quinoa and whole wheat are good sources of protein.

Iron is found in legumes, beans, tofu, spinach and fortified cereals.

Vitamin C can improve iron absorption.

Calcium is found in almonds, tofu, leafy greens and fortified plant milk.

B12 vitamin is found in animal products, so fortified foods like nutritional yeast and plant milk can be beneficial.

Omega-3 fatty acids can be found in plant-based sources like hemp seeds, walnuts, chia seeds and flaxseeds.

Zinc is found in whole grains, beans, lentils, seeds and nuts, also absorption can be improved by soaking, sprouting or fermenting grains and legumes.

Fibre is found in fruits, vegetables, whole grains and legumes.

A balanced meal should include a variety of healthful grains, veggies and protein sources. Seeking personalised guidance from a licensed dietitian or healthcare expert is always a smart idea.

CONCLUSION

Embracing a Veggie and Protein Lifestyle

A veggie and protein lifestyle is a diet primarily based on plant-based foods and protein sources, often associated with vegetarianism or veganism. It can also include flexitarian or pescatarian approaches, where some animal products are consumed.

To adopt this lifestyle, diversify your plant-based foods, explore plant-based protein sources, include whole grains like brown rice, quinoa, bulgur and oats, also snack on nuts and seeds for protein and healthy fats. Experiment with tofu and tempeh in various dishes and explore plant-based dairy alternatives like almond milk, soy milk and coconut yoghurt.

Plan balanced meals with a mix of carbohydrates, proteins and fats for sustained energy. Supplement wisely with vitamin B12, vitamin D and omega-3 fatty acids, as these nutrients are sometimes lacking in plant-based diets.

Try plant-based meat alternatives like veggie burgers, plant-based sausages or meatless meatballs for familiar flavours and textures. Stay informed about your body's nutritional needs and ensure adequate intake of essential nutrients.

Stay hydrated by drinking plenty of water and consider herbal teas or infused water for variety. Listen to your body's signals and consult with a healthcare professional or registered dietitian if you feel fatigued or notice any deficiencies.

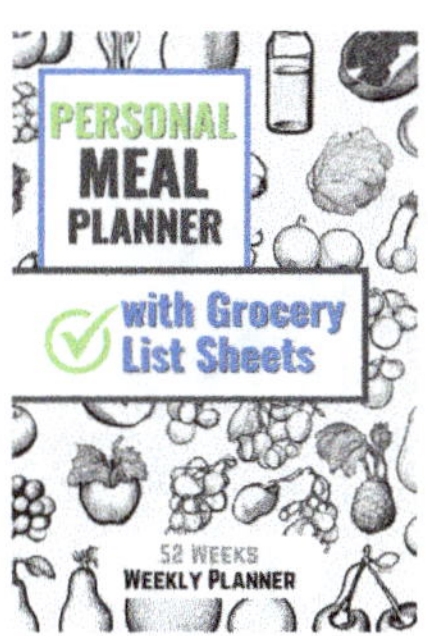

You can also Get Your Personal Meal Planner by visiting the link below:

https://www.amazon.com/dp/B0CTHD4VGR

www.ingramcontent.com/pod-product-compliance
Lightning Source LLC
Chambersburg PA
CBHW080727260726
48660CB00010B/3733